From Belly **Fat**
to Belly **FLAT**

From Belly **Fat** to Belly **FLAT**

The MEDICALLY PROVEN Diet to RESHAPE YOUR BODY

Dr C W Randolph, Jr
author of *From Hormone Hell to Hormone Well*
and **Genie James**

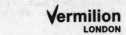

Vermilion
LONDON

1 3 5 7 9 10 8 6 4 2

Published in 2009 by Vermilion, an imprint of Ebury Publishing
Ebury Publishing is a Random House Group company

First published in the United States in 2008 by Health Communications, Inc.

Copyright © C W Randolph, Jr, MD, and Genie James 2008

C W Randolph, Jr, MD, and Genie James have asserted their right to be identified as the
authors of this Work in accordance with the Copyright, Designs and Patents Act 1988.

The Random House Group Limited Reg. No. 954009

Addresses for companies within the Random House Group can be found at
www.rbooks.co.uk

A CIP catalogue record for this book is available from the British Library

The Random House Group Limited supports The Forest Stewardship
Council (FSC), the leading international forest certification organisation.
All our titles that are printed on Greenpeace approved FSC certified paper carry the FSC logo.
Our paper procurement policy can be found at www.rbooks.co.uk/environment

Printed and bound in Great Britain by
CPI Cox & Wyman, Reading, RG1 8EX

ISBN 9780091929565

Text design by Dawn Von Strolley Grove

Copies are available at special rates for bulk orders. Contact the sales development team
on 020 7840 8487 for more information.

To buy books by your favourite authors and register for offers, visit www.rbooks.co.uk

The information in this book has been compiled by way of general guidance in relation
to the specific subjects addressed, but is not a substitute and not to be relied on for medical,
healthcare, pharmaceutical or other professional advice on specific circumstances and in
specific locations. Please consult your GP before changing, stopping or starting any
medical treatment. So far as the author is aware the information given is correct and up to
date as of January 2009. Practice, laws and regulations all change, and the reader should
obtain up to date professional advice on any such issues. The authors and publishers
disclaim, as far as the law allows, any liability arising directly or indirectly from the use,
or misuse, of the information contained in this book.

To John R Lee, MD, my friend, my mentor
and a courageous medical pioneer,
and to my mother, Smiles Randolph,
who always believes in me,
my abilities and my dreams with unconditional faith.

CWR

CONTENTS

ACKNOWLEDGEMENTS

This book would not have become a reality without the input, talent and support of many individuals, including my co-author, Genie James. Before I acknowledge each of them, however, I want to thank God for giving me the inspiration and courage to become both a physician and a healer. I am humbly aware that it is my privilege to serve as an instrument of our Creator. I also want to thank my mother, Smiles Randolph, for always believing in me and encouraging me to speak the truth.

I would not currently be regarded as a medical expert and a pioneer in the realm of bio-identical hormone replacement had it not been for my friend and mentor, the late John R Lee, MD, primary author of *What Your Doctor May Not Tell You About Perimenopause*, *What Your Doctor May Not Tell You About Menopause* and *What Your Doctor May Not Tell You About Breast Cancer*. Dr Lee's fingerprints remain on my heart and in my work.

In the medical and scientific fields, I would like to thank Joel Hargrove, MD, for his willingness to oppose the pharmaceutical industry through his tenacity for groundbreaking medical research in the field of bio-identical hormone replacement; Christiane Northrup, MD, for her unmistakable voice and published works that first helped to introduce the term *bio-identical* into the layperson's vocabulary; Erika Schwartz, MD, for her strength and courage as a spokeswoman for our cause; Helene Leonetti, MD, for research substantiating the clinical benefits of bio-identical progesterone replacement; Joann E Manson, MD, for her work in preventive medicine and hormone replacement; Kenna Stephenson, MD, for her research examining how bio-identical hormone replacement positively influences women's cardiovascular health and ageing process; James L Wilson, ND, for his illuminating work on the adrenal hormones; and David Zava, PhD, for his daring research linking breast cancer and synthetic hormone replacement.

I also want to acknowledge Virginia Hopkins for her pivotal role in working with Dr Lee to co-author the above-mentioned three books, which set the stage for the current revolution supporting the use of bio-identical hormone therapies. Since Dr Lee's death, Ms Hopkins continues her mission to educate the public about the safety and efficacy of bio-identical hormones through her website and newsletter.

Special kudos go to Colleen Reilly, executive director of Women in Balance, for her efforts to provide education on available research and for her willingness to address the confusion that healthcare providers express about hormone therapies – especially since the National Institutes of Health halted the Women's Health Initiative (WHI) study of synthetic hormone replacement therapy in postmenopausal women in July 2002.

Similarly, I applaud the leadership teams at the Professional Compounding Center of America (PCCA) and the International Association of Compounding Pharmacies (IACP) for their stamina in fighting the money-for-power exchange between pharmaceutical lobbyists and members of Congress. I am excited by the strides that these two organisations, along with Jim Paoletti (now at ZRT Laboratories), are making in educating the medical community on the safety and efficacy of bio-identical hormone replacement.

I have true gratitude for Nanette Noffsinger, our media and public relations consultant. Ms Noffsinger represents us with a passion and an integrity that is inspiring. The fact that she could actually convince me to put on face powder before going before a camera is a testament to her gamut of skills!

Thanks are due to Susan Shee, our marketing coordinator and patient liaison for the Natural Hormone Institute of America. For more than a year, she patiently accomplished the day-to-day work, thereby allowing Ms James to focus on this project. Others I would like to thank include John Kaszuba for his cutting-edge marketing talents and his help with our website and newsletter, as well as Mikel Taft and Jessica Vance, for their help typing, formatting and walking the dogs when necessary. I also want to acknowledge Patti Landry, NP, Anna Stauch, NP, and Nicole Avens, NP. Patti gracefully and firmly models the best of mind-body-spirit medicine; Anna blends extreme intelligence with sharp intuition as she cares for patients. Although Nicole is no longer with the practice, I continue to have the greatest admiration for her skills as an integrative medicine provider, particularly in the area of bio-identical hormone replacement. My entire office staff is incredible. It is because of their skills and commitment that we are able to serve a wide range of patients.

Finally, my deepest gratitude goes to my patients. Their weight-loss success stories created the framework for this book.

It has been a privilege to write this book. As a physician and a healer, I have always been grateful to serve one person at a time, but hours and logistics limit how many people one can touch or help in such a role. Thankfully, this book fulfills the mission to meet a wider breadth of need.

Even if you and I never meet or have a one-to-one conversation, perhaps you will embrace our three-step plan and, in doing so, save yourself a lifetime struggle with abdominal weight gain, other symptoms of hormone imbalance and the risk of developing hormone-dependent cancers. Nothing brings me more joy than seeing patients living healthy, happy lives. I wish the same for you.

Dr C W Randolph, Jr

I am indebted to Pat Holdsworth, who evidenced a personal graciousness and tenacity that would ultimately characterise our entire publishing team at Health Communications. Most especially, I express deep thanks to Allison Janse and Michele Matrisciani for believing in the merit of this project and sharing their editing wisdom and enthusiasm for disseminating the truth.

Sincere appreciation also goes to Michelle Howry, now senior editor at Touchstone Fireside, because her input shifted the tone of this book and made it more accessible to the reader. I also thank Laura Yorke of the Carol Mann Agency for her initial contributions, her footwork and her willingness to introduce us to a new realm of publishing.

Genie James

INTRODUCTION: THE LINK BETWEEN OESTROGEN AND BELLY FAT

I f you're a woman over thirty or a man over forty who has gained unwanted weight around your waist and belly, this book is for you. I hope to share information that will eliminate your guilt and feelings of resignation about your weight, and will also provide you with a solution. My premise, which is medically proven, is this: those extra pounds that have crept up and become cemented around your middle have little to do with your inability to diet properly, limit carbs or do crunches; they have everything to do with a shift in hormone production. In fact, belly fat is commonly the outward sign of a specific type of underlying hormone imbalance known as oestrogen dominance.

As long as oestrogen dominance remains unrecognised and untreated, your belly fat will be nearly impossible to lose, no

A Note to Readers: While this book was a team effort, it is written from Dr Randolph's perspective, since he has treated thousands of patients. Through his hands-on experience as a physician, he uncovered the link between oestrogen and belly fat.

matter what you do or how hard you try. Fortunately, oestrogen dominance can be eliminated almost effortlessly and, once hormone balance is restored, the pounds that are attached to your middle will start to melt away without food deprivation or calorie counting.

How do I know this? As a physician, I have focused my life's work on how to safely and effectively reestablish optimal hormonal balance, mostly in women. I graduated from Auburn University's School of Pharmacy in 1971 and worked as a licensed compounding pharmacist before returning to university to become a physician. I received my medical degree from Louisiana State University School of Medicine in 1982 and my board certification in obstetrics and gynaecology in 1986.

Over the past decade, my professional expertise has expanded to include a focus on natural, or integrative, medicine. In 2000, I attended a continuing medical education program at Columbia University Medical School, where I completed intensive training under Andrew Weil, MD. In 2005, I became a board-certified Diplomate of the American Board of Holistic Medicine. It humbles me that after more than two decades of clinical practice, I am internationally recognised as a pioneer in the field of bio-identical hormone replacement therapies (BHRT). *Bio-identical* refers to plant-derived hormone molecules that are identical to the natural human hormones produced by the body.

the cure for the 'bloated belly' syndrome

For years, women have sought my help as a physician because they knew something wasn't right. They came to my office suffering from symptoms such as hot flushes, night sweats, irregular bleeding, bloating, memory loss, low libido and mood swings. In almost every case, these women also evidenced another unwanted side effect: abdominal weight gain. They used all sorts of terms to describe their extra weight: 'protruding tummy', 'bloated belly', 'pregnant stomach', or even 'that new continent that has attached itself to my hips'. Men who realised that something was shifting with their hormones also sought help. Most often, male patients' primary symptoms would be loss of sex drive, fatigue and depression. The fact that these men almost always had a spare tyre was just part of the presenting package.

During the patients' physical examinations, I would most always write 'increased abdominal circumference' on their medical charts. Then, without paying any more attention to their weight, I would move on to address what I considered a more pressing concern: how their health was being sabotaged by shifting hormone production and, subsequently, an underlying condition of oestrogen dominance. I wasn't aware then of the link between hormone levels and the size of a person's waist.

Based on my background in pharmacology and medical training, I developed a holistic approach to treat this condition of oestrogen dominance. The approach has three components:

1. A diet specifically designed to reduce the body's oestrogen levels.
2. Natural hormone replacement therapy to restore hormone equilibrium.
3. A select list of vitamins and supplements that have been proven to work synergistically to support optimal hormone balance.

the results

After following the plan, hormone balance was restored in all of my patients, and their symptoms of oestrogen dominance disappeared. Their overall health improved usually within one or two months. But, surprisingly, within a week or two, most patients enjoyed an additional benefit: those stubborn pounds they carried around for years began to melt away, and their bellies went from bloated to flat! Within several months, many patients came to me, requesting what they called the 'belly-flat diet'.

I soon realised that this plan could help many people beyond the scope of my medical practice. So, I elicited the help of Genie James, the co-author of my first book, *From Hormone Hell to Hormone Well*, the co-founder of the Natural Hormone Institute of America, also my wife. Not only does she have a Masters of Medical Science from Emory University, she has a distinct expertise in the fields of women's health and complementary medicine.

Once we shared the plan publicly, we saw tremendous results. In general, men and women who committed to the diet saw exciting results in just three to four weeks. A typical first-month response was a loss of 4 to 7 pounds (1.8 to 3.2 kilograms). More important, most waistlines shrank by one to two inches (2.5 to 5 centimetres) in the first few weeks.

By the second month, the pounds and inches dropped even faster, because once hormonal equilibrium was reestablished, the body's metabolism picked up and burned even more calories for energy.

And although the primary goal of this book is to eliminate the underlying condition of oestrogen dominance that is causing unwanted weight gain, the benefits of the plan extend beyond the cosmetic; innumerable medical studies also link oestrogen dominance with several potentially lethal health risks.

If you stay on the plan indefinitely, it will have a long-term positive impact on your overall health and well being. It will give you a lifetime of balanced hormones, a flat belly and better health. Is there any reason you should not get started today?

WHERE YOUR BELLY FAT CAME FROM AND WHY IT *WON'T* BUDGE

My guess is that you picked up this book because, over the last few years, you have put on 10, 20, 30 or even 40 extra pounds (4.5, 9, 13.5 or even 18 extra kilograms) around your abdomen, hips and thighs. The extra weight makes you feel uncomfortable and unattractive. You've tried dieting and exercising to lose the belly fat and, while you may have lost a few pounds here and there for short periods of time, the bulk of your extra weight just hangs on.

In Part 1, you'll learn the medical reason why your belly fat appeared and why it just won't budge, no matter how hard you try. In Chapter 1, you'll learn how hormone balance is intricately connected with your body's metabolism and its predisposition to store fat. Even more important, you'll come to understand why oestrogen dominance is very likely the primary hidden culprit adding pounds to your belly and inches to your waist. Already wondering if you might be oestrogen dominant? In Chapter 2, you'll learn how to self-diagnose the problem.

PART

WHERE YOUR BELLY FAT CAME FROM AND WHY IT WON'T BUDGE

OESTROGEN DOMINANCE: THE HIDDEN WEIGHT-GAIN EPIDEMIC

①

When people hear the term *hormonal imbalance*, most immediately think about the change of life, the menopause. Although it's true that women going through the menopause have significant hormonal changes, the issues associated with hormonal imbalance, such as abdominal weight gain, typically begin in a woman's early to mid-thirties and a man's early forties.

In fact, weight-loss research proves that because of shifting hormone production, the average person will add 1 to 2 pounds (450 to 900 grams) around his or her middle each year between the ages of thirty-five and fifty-five. As long as your body's cellular metabolism is compromised by an untreated hormone imbalance – most particularly oestrogen dominance – the extra pounds around your middle will be nearly impossible to lose.

I firmly believe that oestrogen dominance is an epidemic in Western societies. We are ageing, we are constantly exposed to environmental oestrogens and too many of us are over-weight.

Unfortunately, because the pharmaceutical industry has created so much marketing hype about a woman's need for oestrogen replacement as a fountain-of-youth treatment for the menopause, most medical practitioners and healthcare consumers are misinformed and/or confused. The conse-quence for millions of people is that the very real condition of oestrogen dominance is often overlooked or, worse, misdiag-nosed and mistreated. For instance, consider the case of a woman I'll call Sylvia.

Sylvia, a thirty-six-year-old divorced mother of three, came to my office six months after moving to Florida from Oregon. She said that she had gained 25 pounds (11 kilo-grams) in three years and was suffering from what she called the 'love-handle blues'. She was in tears as she explained the following:

Ever since my divorce three years ago, I have felt as if someone was pumping up a spare tyre around my middle. I used to be a size 8, and now I can barely squeeze into a size 12. I swear I'm not eating any more than I did five years ago. If anything, I eat less. Even though I go to the gym and walk on a treadmill at least five hours a week, this fat around my belly just won't budge.

I can't go on this way. I am almost at the point of considering diet pills. Also, my doctor had put me on antidepressants, but my prescription has expired. Please help me.

Sylvia's age, weight gain and mild depression were common indicators of an underlying hormonal imbalance, specifically oestrogen dominance. I told Sylvia that I could help her without diet pills or antidepressants. After following the plan for six weeks, she walked into the office a changed woman. She had lost 9 pounds (4 kilograms) and an inch and a half (4 centimetres) from her waist. Within ten weeks, she celebrated with a shopping spree for new size 10 trousers. In my practice, I have helped thousands of people like Sylvia, people who had no idea that shifting hormone production was the hidden culprit causing their weight gain.

In order for you to understand how a hormone imbalance could affect your weight, here's a quick refresher course in the production and function of your sex hormones.

oestrogen and progesterone: a careful balancing act

The human body produces three sex hormones: oestrogen, progesterone and testosterone. In this book I focus primarily on oestrogen and progesterone because both medical research and my experience prove that they play the starring roles in any hormone-related weight-gain drama.

healthy hormone function from puberty to thirty

When a woman begins to menstruate until she is approximately thirty years old, her ratio of oestrogen to progesterone is optimal. In this ideal scenario, oestrogen does the following for her:

- Develops the sex organs and secondary sex characteristics such as breasts and pubic hair.
- Maintains the menstrual cycle.

- Supports the growth and function of the uterus, specifically creating the lining of the uterus to prepare it for pregnancy.
- Stimulates cell growth.

During these same years, progesterone does the following:

- Maintains the uterus and prepares it for pregnancy during the reproductive years.
- Promotes the survival of an ovum (egg) once it is fertilised.
- Stimulates bone building that can prevent or treat osteoporosis.
- Acts as a natural diuretic to prevent bloating.

In women and men, progesterone also does the following:

- Serves as a natural antidepressant.
- Fosters a calming effect on the body.
- Maintains libido.
- Promotes regular sleep patterns.
- Opposes oestrogen's predisposition to promote cell growth, thereby providing protection from uterine, breast and ovarian cancer as well as fibrocystic disease in females and an increased risk of prostate cancer in males.

As you can see, when they are in sync, oestrogen and progesterone are responsible for important biochemical functions in both the female and male bodies. When the ratio of oestrogen to progesterone gets out of sync, many health issues arise, including unwanted weight gain.

what is oestrogen dominance?

It is important to understand that being oestrogen dominant doesn't mean that your body is producing too much oestrogen; rather, it means that your body's oestrogen production is not balanced by progesterone production. Oestrogen dominance occurs when the natural ratio of oestrogen to progesterone is upset – in other words, when the body's internal oestrogen-to-progesterone seesaw becomes tilted.

a weight-gain double whammy: how your body becomes a 'fat magnet'

Oestrogen dominance causes a host of metabolic disturbances, which occur much like a chicken-and-egg relationship:

- Too much oestrogen circulating in the body increases body fat, and fatty tissue within the body produces and stores more oestrogen. Body fat contains an enzyme that converts adrenal steroids to oestrogen. At a cellular level, body fat continues to produce more oestrogen, and a high oestrogen level, in turn, causes the body to increase its store of fatty tissue. In other words, your belly becomes a 'fat magnet'.
- When you're oestrogen dominant, your body is unable to effectively use fat stores for energy, which means that your body's ability to metabolise or burn body fat for calories is compromised. The result is extra weight that won't go away even with more exercise or less eating.
- When high oestrogen levels are unopposed by sufficient progesterone, the resulting condition of oestrogen

dominance also impacts your body fat's distribution. In both men and women, higher oestrogen levels predispose the body to store fat around the abdomen. In women, oestrogen dominance causes fat to be stored around the waist, hips and thighs, and it's the main reason that many middle-aged women have pearshaped bodies. Oestrogen dominance is also the reason for the middle-aged spare tyre in men.

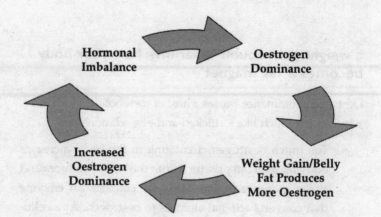

Hormonal Imbalance → **Oestrogen Dominance** → **Weight Gain/Belly Fat Produces More Oestrogen** → **Increased Oestrogen Dominance**

effects on the thyroid gland

The thyroid gland is best known for its metabolic function affecting weight. Oestrogen dominance renders the thyroid hormones dysfunctional, causing your body's metabolism to slow down. The resulting condition is called *relative hypothyroidism*. In addition, the changes in your body's blood sugar levels – some of which occur naturally with age and some of which are due to a hormone imbalance – are also linked to weight gain. As the body's progesterone production decreases with age and oestrogen becomes dominant, your body releases insulin more rapidly and more often. When fluctuating hormones unnaturally stimulate insulin release, you get hungry faster and will often crave sugar. In fact, these food cravings can sometimes be uncontrollable, and people who are oestrogen dominant tend to consume more sweets even when they aren't truly hungry. As a result, they ingest more calories than their bodies require and pack on even more pounds.

If you are a woman in your thirties, you need to understand that oestrogen dominance is not 'your mother's problem'. For most women, oestrogen dominance is a concern to be reckoned with long before middle age or the menopause. As a woman approaches her mid-thirties, the balance of hormones within her body begins to shift, starting with a decline in progesterone. In fact, progesterone production declines 120 times more rapidly than does oestrogen production. It is this downward shift in progesterone production that causes the body to become oestrogen dominant.

Contrary to the popular belief that oestrogen is solely a female hormone, men can also be oestrogen dominant. In men, progesterone is produced in the adrenal and testicular tissue. When men reach their forties, falling progesterone levels lead to a fall in testosterone levels. As both the progesterone and testosterone levels decline, the male body becomes oestrogen dominant. To find out if oestrogen dominance is responsible for your increased belly fat – and possibly a host of other physical, mental and emotional concerns and health risks – continue reading. Chapter 2 will help you to understand how age, body fat and environmental toxins can join forces to sabotage your inner hormonal equilibrium.

ARE YOU OESTROGEN DOMINANT?

Evelyn, a thirty-seven-year-old graphic artist and mother of three, walked into my office literally dragging her forty-three-year-old husband, Richard, behind her. I had delivered all three of her children and had been her gynaecologist for years. Evelyn related the following:

Dr Randolph, remember how trim and athletic my body was even after three kids? Even two years ago, I was a perfect size 10. Now I am a size 14 and I look like I swallowed a bowling ball.

I am still relatively young. I'm not even forty, but I feel like I am living in a stranger's body. And I am not the only one. Until three years ago, he [pointing to Richard] could wear the same golfing gear he wore in college. Now he's gained 30 pounds (14.5 kilograms) in the last four years.

I cook all the same foods I have for the past fifteen years, so I know it's not a change in our diet. I still go to an aerobics class every other morning and play tennis three times a week. So what could it be? Just old age?

11

Evelyn and Richard were both experiencing oestrogen dominance and were exhibiting 'flashing red light' symptoms and behaviours. To determine if you might be oestrogen dominant, answer the four questions below.

OESTROGEN DOMINANCE SELF-ASSESSMENT
❑ Question 1: How Old Are You?

If you are a woman older than thirty or a man older than forty (men, see page 13 for further details), you are most likely oestrogen dominant.

As mentioned in the last chapter, a woman's progesterone level begins to decline in her thirties, even while the ovaries are still producing enough oestrogen to stimulate the monthly cycle. From early or mid-thirties through mid- or late forties, a woman who is regularly menstruating is said to be premenopausal. When a woman's periods become irregular – in some cases skipping months at a time and in other cases becoming heavy and flooding – she is said to be perimenopausal. In this stage of life, the ovaries' production of oestrogen is also declining, but progesterone production continues to decline even more significantly. The result is continual oestrogen dominance.

Even during and after the menopause, oestrogen dominance is still a concern. The average age of a woman entering natural menopause in the United Kingdom is fifty-one years old. Many women make the mistake of thinking that if they are no longer menstruating, they no longer have to worry about the levels of hormones that are circulating in their bodies. This is wrong. It is a misconception to believe that when a woman stops having periods, her ovaries turn off like a light switch.

Although the menopause indicates a drastic shift in your body's hormonal equilibrium, it does not mean that the sex hormones are suddenly absent from your body. The ovaries of a menopausal woman are still quite actively producing 40 to 60 per cent of the oestrogen produced by a premenopausal woman. Progesterone production, however, continues to decline. The result is that many menopausal and post-menopausal women continue to suffer from oestrogen dominance.

Before the age of 55, one in every five women in the UK will enter an abrupt, artificial menopause as the result of a hysterectomy. If you are a woman who has had a partial hysterectomy – that is, removal of the uterus only – you can still be oestrogen dominant because your ovaries will continue to produce some oestrogen and even less progesterone.

If you are a woman who has had a complete hysterectomy – that is, removal of the entire reproductive tract (the uterus, fallopian tubes and ovaries), you can still be oestrogen dominant. Even though you no longer have ovaries, your body fat is still producing oestrogen.

Oestrogen-Dominant Men

For men, *Question 1* is easy. If you are a man older than forty, your progesterone and testosterone levels have already started to decline. If you feel sluggish, bloated and/or lethargic, these are symptoms of an underlying hormonal imbalance. Your age and your symptoms indicate that you are in the midst of the male menopause, or andropause. Decreased sexual appetite, abdominal weight gain and an inability to lose weight are three indications that you are most likely oestrogen dominant.

❑ Question 2: How Long Have You Been Overweight?

If you have been 10 pounds (4.5 kilograms) overweight for a year or more, you are most likely caught in the cycle of increasing oestrogen dominance. As described in Chapter 1, high oestrogen levels cause you to develop more fatty tissue in your body, which in turn produces more oestrogen in your body.

❑ Question 3: Do You Have Symptoms of Oestrogen Dominance?

Weight gain is only one symptom of an underlying hormone imbalance. Because hormone receptors are located throughout the body and in the brain, oestrogen dominance can manifest in a host of physical, emotional and mental ailments. These include anxiety, depression fatigue, breast tenderness, headaches (including migraines), digestive disorders, fuzzy thinking and/or memory loss and low libido. Look at the box on page 15. If two or more of these symptoms apply to you, and if these symptoms have been present for more than three months, it is likely a signal that you are suffering from an underlying condition of oestrogen dominance.

Symptoms of Hormone Imbalance

Women	Men
Mood swings	Burned out feeling
Hot flushes	Abdominal fat
Night sweats	Prostate problems
Fatigue	Decreased mental clarity
Headaches	Decreased sex drive
Depressed	Increased urinary urge
Anxious	Decreased strength
Nervous	Decreased stamina
Irritable	Difficulty sleeping
Tearful	Decreased urine flow
Memory lapse	Irritable
Weight gain	Depressed
Premature ageing	Erectile dysfunction
Vaginal dryness	Night sweats
Heavy periods	Poor concentration
Bleeding changes	
Incontinence	
Fibrocystic breasts	
Decreased sex drive	
Tender breasts	
Osteoporosis	
Water retention	

❏ Question 4: Does Your Environment Put You at Risk?

Simply living in an industrialised nation puts you at risk for oestrogen dominance. However, if you are in a work situation where you are constantly being exposed to toxic fumes or if your home is located near a toxic waste dump, the chances that your environment is contributing to your condition of oestrogen dominance is even greater.

Environmental oestrogen, or xenoestrogen (pronounced 'ZEE-no-oestrogen'), can be found in pesticides, herbicides, fungicides, plastics, fuels, car exhausts, dry cleaning chemicals, industrial waste and meat from animals that have been fed oestrogenic drugs to fatten them. It is also found in the synthetic oestrogen and progesterone (chemically termed *progestin*) of birth control pills and hormone therapies; these synthetic hormones are secreted in women's urine, are flushed down the toilet and eventually make their way back into the food chain. Over time, these foreign oestrogens can dangerously accumulate and increase the oestrogen load in the body.

People living in the United States and in western Europe have been found to have much higher oestrogen levels at much younger ages than people living in less industrialised countries. Many experts link these high levels of oestrogen to environmental exposure. Oestrogen-like hormones in the foods we eat and the chemicals we use every day are often hidden causes of oestrogen dominance. These oestrogen-like hormones mimic the action of the oestrogen produced in our bodies. We are exposed to them through certain chemicals (xenoestrogens) and through specific types of foods and plants (phytoestrogens).

Although most of our exposure to xenoestrogens comes in small amounts, the problem is that most of us are exposed to many tiny doses every day, which has a dangerous, cumulative effect.

Chronic exposure to environmental oestrogens can contribute to oestrogen dominance occurring at a much younger age. The increasing number of younger women who are experiencing anovulatory menstrual cycles is a silent signal of oestrogen dominance. An anovulatory cycle is a cycle in which ovulation fails to occur, which means that a woman bleeds but doesn't release an egg, or ovulate. Anovulatory cycles occur when a woman's body isn't making enough progesterone to balance the oestrogen that builds up the uterine lining. Medical studies have shown that by age thirty-five, approximately 50 per cent of women are having anovulatory cycles.

Even women and men in their teens and twenties have been found to suffer from oestrogen dominance that stems from environmental exposure. The symptoms include weight gain, PMT, fibrocystic breasts, bloating, troublesome periods, infertility, endometriosis, depression and mood swings.

Xenoestrogens

Xeno literally means foreign; therefore, xenoestrogens are foreign oestrogens. In addition to being highly oestrogenic, xenoestrogens are fat soluble and nonbiodegradable. This means that they easily pass through the skin and sit in fatty tissues and that they don't break down over time, in either the body or the environment. Some common sources of xenoestrogens include:

Meat and dairy products. In the United States, most ranchers inject their cattle and sheep with synthetic steroid growth-promoting hormones. Growth-promoting hormone implants have been banned in the EU since 1988. The UK government introduced its own ban in December 1986.

Pesticides and plastics. Chemical pesticides, herbicides and fungicides are routinely applied to mass-produced fruit and vegetables. In addition, most people routinely use bug sprays, weed killers and other pesticides in their homes and gardens. Finally, plastic products are part of almost every person's daily life, and many of them give off xenoestrogens when heated, whether purposely in a microwave or accidentally in a hot car.

Petrochemicals and solvents. Many general hygiene products – such as skin cream, lotion, soap, shampoo, perfume, hair spray and air fresheners – contain petrochemicals. These compounds often have chemical structures similar to oestrogen and therefore act like oestrogen when introduced into the body. Industrial solvents are another source of xenoestrogens and are commonly found in cosmetics, nail polish, nail polish remover, glue, paint, varnish, cleaning products, carpet, fibreboard and other processed woods.

Synthetic hormone replacement drugs and birth control pills. Synthetic hormone replacement drugs such as Prematrin, Preminque and Kliovance and many other brand names, as well as birth control pills, contribute to the development or worsening of oestrogen dominance.

Many doctors routinely continue to prescribe synthetic hormone replacement therapy for menopausal symptoms, such as hot flushes, night sweats, insomnia and moodiness. These prescription drugs are composed of synthetic oestrogen or a synthetic oestrogen and progestin combination. Synthetic hormone replacement has also been prescribed to protect women from the loss of bone mass after the menopause.

More than a decade ago, we became convinced that natural bio-identical hormone replacement therapy (BHRT) was a safer and more effective option for treating the symptoms of hormone imbalance than synthetic hormones manufactured and marketed by large pharmaceutical companies. In fact, our first book, *From Hormone Hell to Hormone Well*, focused on the benefits of BHRT versus synthetic hormone therapies. (BHRT is available on prescription privately in the UK.)

Like synthetic hormone replacement pills, birth control pills also contain synthetic oestrogen and progestin. Depending on dosage, they can be very potent and linger in the body for a long time. Birth control pills work by keeping oestrogen at such a falsely high level that the body is fooled into responding as if it were pregnant. Therefore, ovulation does not occur. Chapter 3 addresses the dangers of synthetic hormones in greater detail.

why the symptoms are often misdiagnosed

When Sylvia in Chapter 1 first complained of the 'love-handle blues', her previous doctor responded by giving her a prescription for antidepressants. Unfortunately, the inappropriate use of antidepressants to treat oestrogen dominance is far too common. In recent years in American, more than 70 per cent of the prescriptions written for the type of anti-depressant called selective serotonin reuptake inhibitors (SSRIs) came from physicians who had no special training in mental health disorders!

It saddens me to realise that many women (and men) who tell their physicians that they suffer from moodiness and mild depression leave their doctor's surgery with a prescription for an antidepressant while their underlying condition of oestrogen dominance remains unrecognised and untreated. Unlike antidepressant drugs or manufactured synthetic hormones, bio-identical hormone therapies cannot be patented. Therefore, there are no company sales repre-sentatives going into physicians' offices to educate them about the causes and dangers of oestrogen dominance.

Because of this ignorance within the medical community, many women and men continue to suffer needlessly. Worst of all, when a woman complains of even the slightest symptoms of oestrogen dominance, most conventional medical doctors recommend a prescription of synthetic oestrogen replace-ment. This practice is both irresponsible and dangerous, and even though it is usually rooted in ignorance, it can have tragic consequences.

the long-term health risks of oestrogen dominance

The relationship between oestrogen dominance and weight gain is a very real concern, but there are others as well. Clinical studies conducted in both the United States and

Europe link oestrogen dominance to many other health risks. For instance, in both men and women, oestrogen-related belly fat is a contributing risk factor for developing cardio-vascular disease. According to the Food and Drug Administration (FDA) in the United States, women with a waist measurement of more than thirty-five inches (89 centimetres) and men with a waist measurement of more than forty inches (102 centimetres) are very likely to be at risk.

Oestrogen also fuels cell growth, and unchecked cell growth, or proliferation, is a precursor for cancer. In women, elevated oestrogen levels have been linked to an increased risk for endometriosis and fibroids as well as breast and uter-ine hormone-dependent cancers. (In hormone-dependent cancers, a tumour requires hormones, specifically oestrogen, in order to grow. The medical term for such tumors is *oestro-gen receptor-positive*.) In men, oestrogen dominance has been linked to an increased risk of hormone-dependent prostate cancer.

An increasing number of studies link exposure to environ-mental oestrogens to an increased risk of cancer. In her book *The Truth About Breast Cancer*, Claire Hoy states the following:

> *Greenpeace found that one country that banned pesticides –*
> *Israel – quickly went from breast cancer rates that were among*
> *the highest in the world to rates in keeping with other indus-*
> *trialised nations. It also found that US counties with chemical*
> *waste sites were 6.5 times more likely to have elevated breast*
> *cancer rates than those without waste sites.*

After reading this chapter, you should be able to determine if your age, your body fat, your symptoms and your chronic exposure to environmental oestrogens signal that you are suffering from oestrogen dominance. If your situation and symptoms fit, then stop feeling guilty about those extra pounds around your middle. They are not your fault. At a cellular level, you have been, and continue to be, set up.

Nevertheless, don't give up. You can eliminate your condition of oestrogen dominance once and for all while having a very positive impact on your overall health and well being. The next few chapters will tell you exactly how.

PART 2

THE THREE-STEP PLAN TO BALANCE YOUR *HORMONES* AND WHITTLE YOUR MIDDLE

The next three chapters will provide you with the details of the three-step plan to balance your hormones and help you acquire the flat belly that goes with it. Chapter 3 describes the foods that will help to decrease your body's oestrogen load. Chapter 4 explains how to safely and effectively boost your body's declining progesterone levels without a prescription. Chapter 5 provides a list of supplements you can take to support overall hormone balance.

STEP 1:
EAT FOODS THAT BALANCE
YOUR HORMONES

A complaint I hear many times a day is 'I try to eat a low-calorie, low-fat diet and I exercise regularly, but no matter what I do, those pounds around my middle just won't budge.' Does this sound familiar?

With an awareness of how certain foods can help to decrease the body's oestrogen load, we have developed a diet, moderately high in calories, that allows for protein and healthy fats at every meal. It includes ample portions of 'belly-blaster' foods that will reduce or eliminate your extra oestrogen load.

THE NON-NEGOTIABLE FOOD LIST: FOODS THAT REDUCE OESTROGEN DOMINANCE

The stars of the nutritional component of the plan are cruciferous vegetables, citrus fruit, insoluble fibre and lignans, because these foods function within your body to reduce an unhealthy oestrogen load.

Belly Blaster 1: Cruciferous Vegetables
Benefit to your body: indole-3-carbinol (I3C)
✓ EAT 2–3 SERVINGS PER DAY.

Cruciferous vegetables are a critical part of your success on this plan. Eating large amounts of broccoli, asparagus, cauliflower, spinach, Brussels sprouts, celery, beetroot, kale, cabbage, parsley root (Hamburg parsley), radish, turnip, spring greens and mustard greens have been shown to improve the production of 'good' oestrogen. Although not considered cruciferous, asparagus and spinach are also 'belly blasters' because they also improve 'good' oestrogen levels.

There are three kinds of natural oestrogens: oestrone (E1), oestradiol (E2) and oestriol (E3). All oestrogens tend to promote cell division, but unchecked cell division can lead to cancer. E2 is the most stimulating to breast and uterine tissues, and E1 is less so; thus, they might be called the 'bad' oestrogens. In contrast, E3 may be thought of as the 'good' oestrogen because medical studies have shown that it protects us from cancer. Cruciferous vegetables contain a phytonutrient called indole-3-carbinol (I3C), which has been shown to act as a catalyst to decrease the body's load of 'bad' oestrogens. These vegetables therefore help to reduce oestrogen dominance.

If you're not a fan of cruciferous vegetables, try some of the recipes in Chapter 8. You just might become a cauliflower convert!

Belly Blaster 2: Citrus Fruit
Benefit to your body: d-Limonene
✓ EAT 1 SERVING PER DAY.

A substance called d-Limonene, which is found in the oils of citrus fruit, has been shown to promote the detoxification of oestrogen. Common citrus fruit are oranges, grapefruit, tangerines, lemons, limes and pomelos. Research has also found that when male and female lab mice were administered an extract of d-Limonene, they lost weight.

Belly Blaster 3: Insoluble Fibre
Benefit to your body: oestrogen binder
✓ EAT 2 SERVINGS PER DAY.

There are two types of fibre: soluble and insoluble. Soluble fibre dissolves in water and is degraded by bacteria in your colon. It forms a gel in your intestines that regulates the flow of waste material through your digestive tract. This type of fibre is found in oatmeal, oat bran, dried peas, beans, lentils, apples, pears, strawberries and blueberries. Soluble fibre is good for you, but no matter how much of it you eat, it won't influence your hormonal equilibrium. Insoluble fibre, on the other hand, can directly help to decrease oestrogen overload. It binds itself to extra oestrogen in the digestive tract, which is then excreted by the body. Sources of insoluble fibre are any whole grains – wholemeal bread, barley, couscous, brown rice, whole-grain cereal and wheat bran – as well as seeds, carrots, cucumbers, courgettes, celery and tomatoes.

Belly Blaster 4: Lignans
Benefit to your body: oestrogen binder
✓ EAT 2–3 TABLESPOONS PER DAY.

Ground or milled flaxseed, sesame seeds and flaxseed oil are part of a food group called *lignans*. The friendly bacteria in our intestines convert plant lignans into a substance that has a weak oestrogen-like activity. When there are low oestrogen levels in your body, these weak lignan oestrogens make up for some of the deficiency. When the body is oestrogen dominant, however, these lignan oestrogens bind to your body's oestrogen receptors, thereby reducing human oestrogen activity at a cellular level.

You can get your daily lignan benefit by adding the above mentioned foods to smoothies, yoghurt or salads. Sesame seed oil (tahini) also makes a delicious salad dressing when mixed with lemon juice, garlic and water in a blender.

Table 3-1 opposite gives a list of the four belly-blasting food groups and recommended daily amounts.

Table 3-1. Foods That Reduce Your Oestrogen Load

Food Group	Servings/Day	Comments
CRUCIFEROUS VEGETABLES (75 g/2¾ oz COOKED) ❖ Broccoli ❖ Rocket ❖ Cauliflower ❖ Brussels sprouts ❖ Celery ❖ Beetroot ❖ Kale ❖ Cabbage ❖ Parsley root (Hamburg parsley) ❖ Radish ❖ Turnip, spring or mustard greens ❖ Bok choi ❖ Swede ❖ Asparagus ❖ Spinach	2–3	Cruciferous vegetables should be cooked by steaming, stir-frying, baking or boiling. Raw cruciferous vegetables contain thyroid inhibitors known as *goitrogens.* Eating excessive amounts of raw cruciferous vegetables has been linked to hypothyroid disease. If you want to eat cruciferous vegetables raw, limit to 2–3 servings per week.
CITRUS FRUIT ❖ 1 medium orange ❖ ½ grapefruit ❖ 2 tangerines ❖ 1–2 pomelos ❖ 2 lemons ❖ 2 limes	1	For a single serving, you may substitute 175 ml/10 fl oz of 100% fruit juice once every other day.

from belly fat to belly flat

Table 3-1. Foods That Reduce Your Oestrogen Load (cont'd)

Food Group	Servings/Day	Comments
INSOLUBLE FIBRE ❖ 100 g (3½ oz) cooked whole grains or wholemeal pasta ❖ 1 slice wholemeal bread ❖ 100 g (3½ oz) cooked barley ❖ 100 g (3½ oz) cooked couscous ❖ 100 g (3½ oz) cooked brown rice ❖ 70 g (2½ oz) whole-grain cereal, such as kasha ❖ 100 g (3½ oz) wheat bran ❖ 30 g (1 oz) pumpkin seeds ❖ 70 g (2½ oz) cooked carrots or 125 g (4½ oz) raw carrots ❖ 100 g (3½ oz) sliced cucumbers ❖ 90 g (3¼ oz) cooked courgette ❖ 125 g (4½ oz) raw celery ❖ 1 medium tomato	2	Read the labels. Some products with 'wholemeal' on the label will be made not with whole grains but with white flour and caramel colouring. Many people make the mistake of thinking that whole-grain products are fattening. They are not unless you add butter or creamy toppings. Leave these off. Healthier seasoning alternatives will be provided in the recipes.
LIGNANS ❖ Flaxseed or sesame seeds ❖ Flaxseed oil	2–3 tablespoons	Stir into low-fat yoghurt or cottage cheese or sprinkle atop steamed vegetables.

OTHER FOODS TO ADD TO YOUR DIET EVERY DAY

A unique feature of this diet is that the food groups work in concert to support optimal hormonal equilibrium, provide energy and promote good health as the pounds melt away. In addition to the belly-blasting foods, you should add the following foods to your daily diet.

Protein

✓ EAT 1 SERVING WITH EVERY MEAL.

Your body needs protein every day. Protein contains the essential amino acids that are required by the body for growth and for the maintenance of lean muscle tissue. In addition, according to a study published in the *Journal of Cell Metabolism*, a high-protein diet can also increase the amount of a hunger-fighting hormone circulating within the body. The hormone, known as peptide YY (or PYY), had already been found by the researchers to reduce food intake by a third when it was administered by injection to both normal-weight and obese people.

Rachel Batterham, the clinical scientist who led the study, said, 'We've now found that increasing the protein content of the diet augments the body's own PYY, helping to reduce hunger and aid weight loss.'

High-protein foods slow the movement of food from the stomach to the intestines. Slower stomach emptying means that you feel full longer and get hungrier later. In addition, protein has a gentle, steady effect on blood sugar, as opposed to the quick, steep rise in blood sugar caused by carbohydrates like white bread, biscuits or a jacket potato. Finally, the body uses more energy (i.e., calories) to digest protein than it does to digest fat or carbohydrates.

Fish is a great source of protein. Salmon, trout, herring, water-packed tuna and mackerel are also excellent sources of omega-3 fatty acids, which medical studies have found to have a strong cardiovascular benefit. Due to the health hazards associated with xenoestrogens that were mentioned in Chapter 2, we urge you to eat only organic meats and poultry, which are produced without chemicals or growth hormones.

Even with organic meats, some choices are better sources of protein than others. Red meat is usually higher in fat, particularly saturated fat. There are, however, plenty of lean complete proteins, including the breast meat of poultry and eggs from organic, free-range hens.

Organic plant sources of protein such as beans, legumes and nuts are also excellent choices, but plant proteins must be combined in order to form a complete protein (e.g., rice and beans).

You should eat a serving of protein with every meal. Table 3-2 below lists some good protein sources.

Table 3-2. Protein Sources and Serving Sizes

Protein Source	Serving Size	Comments
Fish	175 g (6 oz)	Steam, bake, grill or stir-fry in olive oil. Do not fry.
Poultry	175 g (6 oz)	Skinless breast meat has the lowest fat.
Eggs	1 large	Boil, scramble or poach.
Black beans	175 g (6 oz)	Combine with rice for a complete protein.
Veggie burger	1 patty	(See recipe in Chapter 8.)
Chickpeas	240 g (8½ oz)	Buy canned and heat, or soak dry chickpeas for 24 hours before cooking.
Dried beans: butter beans, black-eyed beans, lentils	190 g (6¾ oz)	Buy canned and heat, or soak dry beans for 24 hours before cooking.
Tree nuts: almonds, pecans, walnuts, Brazil nuts	35 g (1¼ oz)	Best raw or roasted. Avoid heavily salted or honey-roasted nuts.
Lean red meats	115 g (4 oz)	Limit to once per week.

Calcium

✓ EAT 2 SERVINGS EVERY DAY.

The body's need for calcium becomes increasingly pertinent for women and men as they age. Human bones replace about one-fifth of their total calcium each year, and there is a constant movement of calcium in and out of the bones, both for repair and to maintain a constant level of calcium in the blood and in other body fluids.

A big bonus for the premenopausal or perimenopausal woman is that calcium has been shown to reduce the abdominal cramping and the muscular contractions that result from PMT. Calcium is even more important for women who are approaching the menopause or who are in the midst of it, because calcium helps to put the brakes on the development of osteoporosis, a debilitating bone disorder that causes brittle bones and a bent or stooped stance. Osteoporosis is a virtual epidemic among British women past the age of fifty, and it results from the body having insufficient calcium.

Men, too, need calcium. The body, regardless of gender, requires a certain amount of calcium to flow through its blood and soft tissues every day in order for the muscles to contract correctly, the blood to clot and the nerves to carry messages. When men don't get adequate amounts of dietary calcium, their bodies meet their calcium needs by stealing the mineral from their bones. This weakens the bones over time and contributes to the development of osteoporosis. Although most people think of calcium deficiency as a woman's problem, one in three women and one in 12 men in the UK will suffer a fracture of the hip, wrist or spine as a result of osteoporosis.

Dairy products are not your only possible source of necessary calcium. The foods shown in Table 3-3 opposite are good sources of calcium.

Table 3-3. Calcium Sources: Serving Sizes

Food	Amount	Calcium
Yoghurt, natural, low-fat	225 g (8 oz)	415
Spring greens, fresh or frozen, steamed or boiled	190 g (6¾ oz)	357
Skimmed milk	225 ml (8 fl oz)	306
Spinach, fresh or frozen, steamed or boiled	180 g (6½ oz)	291
Cheese	25 g (1 oz)	162
Cottage cheese, low-fat	225 g (8 oz)	138
Baked beans, canned	250 g (9 oz)	154
Cos or looseleaf lettuce	1 head	97
Canned salmon	85 g (3 oz)	181
Oranges	175 g (6 oz)	72
Almonds	25 g (1 oz)	70
Black-eyed beans, boiled	190 g (6¾ oz)	211
Green peas, boiled	115 g (4 oz)	94

While I recommend that adult women and men consume between 1,200 and 1,500 milligrams (mg) of calcium per day, it is difficult to achieve this goal without supplementation. I will address calcium supplements later in this chapter.

Fruits

✓ EAT 1 SERVING EACH DAY.

Fruit are an important source of fibre, and they are also low in fat and sodium while containing antioxidants and vitamins that contribute to your health. Reach first for colour-rich fruit such as blueberries or strawberries.

I recommend the following single serving of fruit each day: (70 g/2½ oz) of berries; one medium apple, pear, peach or banana; or one medium avocado.

Healthy Oils

✓ USE AS NEEDED IN COOKING OR AS A CONDIMENT.

For cooking and salad dressings, you can use extra-virgin olive oil. In addition to providing a delicious flavouring to cooked foods and salads, olive oil has been shown in studies to have a heart-protective benefit. Other healthy oils include rapeseed oil and flaxseed oil. However, because flaxseed oil is heat sensitive, do not use for cooking. Use flaxseed oil for making salad dressings or mixing in yoghurt or smoothies.

In contrast, avoid cooking with or consuming margarine, butter and corn, sunflower, safflower or peanut oil, as they have been found to promote heart and vascular disease.

Beverages

✓ DRINK EIGHT GLASSES EACH DAY.

Very simply, drink water – lots of it, six to eight glasses a day (1.2 litres). Drink a glass of water with each meal and then sip throughout the rest of the day. Although water contains no calories and might not contain any micronutrients, it is an indispensable aid to digestion, nutrient absorption and waste elimination. Add the juice of half a lemon or lime whenever possible; fresh lemon or lime juice relieves symptoms of indigestion such as heartburn, bloating and belching. Drinking lemon or lime juice regularly aids the bowels in eliminating waste more efficiently, thus controlling constipation and diarrhoea. In addition, there is a belief in Ayurvedic medicine (an ancient system of healthcare native to India) that a cup of hot water with lemon juice in it tones and purifies the liver. Water also impacts how your body metabolises fat. One of the functions of the liver is to convert stored fat to energy; another is to support kidney function. According to Maia Appleby, author of 'Why Drinking Water Really Is the Key to Weight Loss':

If the kidneys are water-deprived, the liver has to do their work along with its own, lowering its total productivity. It then can't metabolize fat as quickly or efficiently as it could when the kidneys were pulling their own weight. If you allow this to happen, not only are you being unfair to your liver, but you're also setting yourself up to store fat.

BELLY-BLASTING DAILY FOOD LIST

Here, for your easy reference, are the recommended foods in their optimum amounts.

Cruciferous vegetables: 2–3 servings a day

Citrus fruit: 1 serving a day

Insoluble fibre: 2 servings a day

Lignans: 2–3 tablespoons a day

Protein: 1 serving with each meal

Calcium: 2 servings a day

Fruit: 1 serving a day (in addition to the citrus)

Healthy oils: as a condiment

Beverages: 8 glasses of water a day

DANGER ZONE: FOODS AND DRINKS THAT INCREASE OESTROGEN LEVELS

Now that you know what foods will decrease your oestrogen load and support hormone balance, we want to help you to avoid consuming foods and drinks that can sabotage everything you are doing to lose weight. When it comes to belly fat, the foods and beverages below are the top five spare-tyre inflators.

Foods high in saturated fats. These foods have been linked to higher levels of oestrogen circulating within the blood. The diet we have recommended therefore excludes the consumption of high-fat meats such as pork sausage, spare ribs, bologna, liverwurst, pork, bacon, ham, frankfurters and bratwurst, as well as commercial salad dressings, chips, crisps, butter, margarine, lard, the shortening in most biscuits and pastries and cream.

Simple carbohydrates. Excessive consumption of refined foods (i.e., the white group) such as sugar, white flour and white rice has been found to raise blood sugar levels and stimulate insulin release, which then negatively impacts hormone balance. Therefore, this diet does not allow refined or processed foods.

Caffeine. Studies have shown that drinking two cups of coffee a day can increase oestrogen levels. In a clinical trial involving approximately 500 women between the ages of thirty-six and forty-five, women who consumed more than one cup of coffee a day had significantly higher levels of oestrogen during the early follicular phase of their menstrual cycle. Those who consumed at least 500 mg of caffeine daily, the equivalent of four or five cups of coffee, had nearly 70 per cent more oestrogen than women who consumed less than 100 mg of caffeine daily. This is why we recommend that you avoid caffeinated products as much as possible, including coffee, caffeinated teas and caffeinated fizzy drinks.

Alcohol. Oestrogen is broken down in the liver. If your liver is diseased or overtaxed, it will be unable to efficiently and effectively break down the oestrogen circulating in your body. According to the American Liver Association and the American Liver Foundation, liver damage can occur when you consume two drinks a day on a daily basis or five to seven drinks a day on the weekend. Because the liver can heal itself by regenerating damaged tissue, abstinence from alcohol can cause a complete reversal and cure without leaving any residual scarring. How long this will take depends on the degree of liver damage.

Phytoestrogens. Phytoestrogens are naturally occurring oestrogenic compounds that are found in a variety of herbs and spices, such as red clover, black cohosh, chasteberry and dong quai. Some of the strongest phytoestrogen-containing foods are soya products, including soyabeans, soya milk, tofu, tempeh, textured vegetable protein, roasted soyabeans, soya granules, miso and edamame. Although their chemical structure resembles oestrogen, it is much less powerful than human oestrogen; in fact, its effectiveness is just a thousandth of human oestrogen's effectiveness. Unlike lignans, which attach to oestrogen and help to reduce oestrogen overload through excretion, soya products actually have the potential to compound the problem.

Consumed in moderation, soya products can be healthy food choices for some people. Nevertheless, for the overweight woman or man with a preexisting condition of oestrogen dominance, eating too much soya can compound an underlying hormone imbalance. Also, nutritional researchers have identified that in some cases soya products act as a potent anti-thyroid agent, suppressing thyroid function and causing or worsening hypothyroidism. Because soya products have the potential to be counterproductive to efforts to eliminate oestrogen dominance, we recommend eliminating all soya products and other phytoestrogens from your diet. We have found that most people don't miss soya products and can easily find many enjoyable alternatives.

the oops, uh-oh factor: when you just can't say no

Over the years, a number of patients have literally started backing out the door the moment they learned that a hormone-balancing diet required them to avoid all caffeine and alcohol. Although zero consumption of these beverages is ideal for maintaining optimal hormonal balance, if you're one of the women or men who can't imagine your morning without a cup of java or your evening without a toddy, we would not want you to walk away from the plan.

In other words, don't throw out the baby with the bathwater. Do your best. If you don't believe you could possibly give up these beverages, just try to limit your consumption to one cup of coffee in the morning and/or one alcoholic beverage (preferably red wine) in the evening. Although red wine will still tax the liver, research indicates that moderate consumption of red wine might help to protect you from heart disease and can have a positive effect on cholesterol levels and blood pressure.

If you do drink any alcohol, try eating a small fibre-rich snack – such as a piece of fruit or half a cup (15 g/½ oz) of whole-grain cereal with skimmed milk – with a bit of protein, like a bite of chicken or salmon. The food will slow the absorption of the alcohol, so it might help you to avoid a quick buzz and an impulsive order of chips with mayonnaise. Then, after one alcoholic drink, order something nonalcoholic and pace yourself.

Finally, if you can't give up your toddies, take milk thistle

as a supplement. Medical studies have shown that milk thistle has a protective effect on the liver and will improve its
function. We recommend taking a 200-mg milk thistle capsule
twice a day.

However, be aware that milk thistle can produce allergic
reactions; these tend to be more common among people who
are allergic to plants in the same family, such as ragweed,
chrysanthemum, marigold and daisy.

Indulging in these habits will slow down your weight-loss
progress a bit, but even small steps will improve your health
and your waistline. Ultimately, only you can decide what you
are willing to give up in order to lose belly fat.

A MONTH OF
HORMONE-BALANCING MEAL PLANS

Instead of obsessing over how many calories you consume,
you should focus on eating foods that reduce your oestrogen
load and support overall hormone balance. Some people like
to keep it simple and eat the same foods every day. For
instance, a patient named Cynthia has stuck to the meal plan
below for nine years.

BREAKFAST: 1 boiled or poached egg, ½ grapefruit, 1 piece of
granary toast with ½ teaspoon of all-fruit natural jam and hot
water with the juice of ½ a lemon.

LUNCH: 175 g (6 oz) of barbecued or grilled chicken breast
marinated in orange juice and low-sodium soya sauce,
steamed broccoli or asparagus, vinegar-marinated coleslaw
and water with lemon.

SNACK: 15 g (4 oz) of low-fat cottage cheese or 300 g (10½ oz) of natural low-fat yoghurt with berries and 2 tablespoons of milled flaxseed.

DINNER: 175 g (6 oz) of grilled fish, spinach salad, steamed cauliflower, brown rice and water with lemon.

Cynthia continues to be a svelte size 10, so if what works for her works for you, go for it. Most people, however, prefer a bit more variety. As a result, we have developed the following month of sample meal plans. Every day includes tasty new ideas for cooking and serving each of the belly-blasting foods groups. We assure you that if you eat the following three meals a day for a month, you will enjoy each meal, you won't walk around hungry and you will lose belly fat and inches.

If a dish is followed by an asterisk (*), its recipe can be found in Chapter 8.

DAY 1

BREAKFAST

1 egg scrambled in olive oil. Sprinkle liberally with dill, dried Italian
  seasoning or 1 tablespoon of fresh salsa, if desired.
1 slice toasted granary bread; spread with 1 teaspoon of all fruit jam
  or butter substitute if desired.
1 small orange
Hot water with the juice of ½ lemon, or herbal tea

LUNCH

Savoury Spinach and Salmon Salad*
Grated Beetroot Salad*
Water with lemon

SNACK

1 medium apple or pear

DINNER

Baked Fish with Basil*
Broccoli or Asparagus with Sesame Seeds*
Mashed Cauliflower*
Water with lemon

DAY 2

BREAKFAST
70 g (2½ oz) whole-grain or bran cereal with 2 tablespoons ground
   flaxseed, 70 g (2½ oz) fresh berries and 225 ml (8 fl oz) skimmed
   milk
1 boiled egg
Hot water with juice of ½ lemon, or herbal tea

LUNCH
170 g (6 oz) sliced turkey or chicken breast
Marinated Broccoli, Cucumber and Tomato Salad*
25 g (1 oz) low-fat cheese
Water with lemon

SNACK
35 g (1¼ oz) almonds or 70 g (2½ oz) pumpkin seeds

DINNER
Lentil, Carrot and Turnip Stew*
Grapefruit and Avocado Salad*
1 slice granary bread
Water with lemon

DAY 3

BREAKFAST
170 g (6 oz) grilled or poached salmon, or 1 egg, poached, soft-boiled, boiled or scrambled
Yoghurt and Fruit Parfait*
Hot water with juice of ½ lemon, or herbal tea

LUNCH
Veggie Burger*
Best Baked Beans*
Cabbage-Apple Salad*
Water with lemon

SNACK
6 celery and carrot sticks
Ginger-Lime Dressing* for dipping

DINNER
175 g (6 oz) Rosemary-Baked Chicken Breast*
Steamed Brussels sprouts tossed with ground or milled flaxseed
Baked Swede*
Water with lemon

DAY 4

BREAKFAST
Asparagus Omelette*
2 slices turkey bacon
125 ml (4 fl oz) grapefruit or orange juice
Hot water with juice of ½ lemon, or herbal tea

LUNCH
Not Your Ordinary Tuna Salad*
50 g (1¾ oz) marinated cauliflower and cherry tomatoes on a bed of
    fresh spinach
Water with lemon

SNACK
Banana in Bark*

DINNER
Grilled 125 g (4 oz) fillet of lean beef
75 g (2¾ oz) steamed broccoli tossed with sesame seeds
Cruciferous Couscous*
Water with lemon

DAY 5

BREAKFAST

1 poached egg
½ grapefruit
1 slice toasted granary bread
Hot water with juice of ½ lemon, or herbal tea

LUNCH

Chicken and Asparagus Lettuce Wraps*
1 medium apple or pear
Water with lemon

SNACK

115 g (4 oz) low-fat cottage cheese, mixed with mandarin orange
   slices and 2 tablespoons ground or milled flaxseed

DINNER

Fish with Citrus Marinade*
Simple Greens and Garlic*
100 g (3½ oz) brown rice; may cook in organic chicken, beef or
   vegetable broth for flavour
Water with lemon

DAY 6

BREAKFAST

150 g (5½ oz) natural yoghurt, mixed with 30 g (1 oz) chopped apple
and 2 tablespoons ground or milled flaxseed. Add ¼ teaspoon of
raw honey and/or cinnamon or nutmeg to taste if desired.

2 rashers back bacon or turkey bacon

Hot water with juice of ½ lemon, or herbal tea

LUNCH

Cauliflower and Turkey Bacon Soup*

Simple Cheese on Toast*

Water with lemon

SNACK

35 g (1¼ oz) almonds or 70 g (2½ oz) pumpkin seeds

DINNER

Pan-Roasted Fish with Parsley and Bacon*

Broccoli or Asparagus with Sesame Seeds*

75 g (2¾ oz) steamed carrots

Water with lemon

DAY 7

BREAKFAST

70 g (2½ oz) whole-grain or bran cereal with 2 tablespoons ground or
    milled flaxseed, 70 g (2½ oz) fresh berries and 225 ml (8 fl oz)
    skimmed milk
1 boiled egg
Hot water with juice of ½ lemon, or herbal tea

LUNCH

Favourite Chicken Salad*
Easy Pickled Beetroots*
Water with lemon

SNACK

1 medium orange or 2 tangerines

DINNER

Quick Turkey-Stuffed Cabbage*
25 g (1 oz) low-fat cheese
Water with lemon

DAY 8

BREAKFAST
2 rashers turkey bacon
1 slice toasted granary bread
½ grapefruit
Hot water with juice of ½ lemon, or herbal tea

LUNCH
Spicy Kale and Beans*
1 sliced cucumber and 1 sliced tomato with salt, pepper, Italian
    seasonings and olive oil or rice wine vinegar
Water with lemon

SNACK
35 g (1¼ oz) almonds or 70 g (2½ oz) pumpkin seeds

DINNER
Lemon Hot Fish*
Asparagus with Sesame Seeds*
55 g (2 oz) wholemeal pasta
Water with lemon

DAY 9

BREAKFAST
Flaxseed and Fruit Smoothie*
175 g (6 oz) poached or grilled salmon
Hot water with juice of ½ lemon, or herbal tea

LUNCH
Veggie Burger* patty (no bun)
Sauerkraut Salad*
1 medium apple or pear
Water with lemon

SNACK
150 g (5½ oz) natural low-fat yoghurt, mixed with 1 tablespoon orange
    juice concentrate, 1 medium orange and 2 tablespoons ground or
    milled flaxseed

DINNER
175 (6 oz) baked, grilled or barbecued chicken breast; marinate in
    orange juice or fat-free Italian dressing if desired.
Indian-Style Brussels Sprouts*
90 g (3¼ oz) steamed yellow squash
1 slice toasted granary bread; spread with butter substitute if desired.
Water with lemon

DAY 10

BREAKFAST
1 poached or boiled egg
Banana in Bark*
Hot water with juice of ½ lemon, or herbal tea

LUNCH
Chicken and Cold Rice Salad*
Easy Pickled Beetroot*
Water with lemon

SNACK
225 ml (8 fl oz) skimmed milk or 300 g (10½ oz) natural low-fat
    yoghurt (add cinnamon or nutmeg if desired) and 70 g (2½ oz)
    berries with 2 tablespoons ground or milled flaxseed

DINNER
Black Beanofritos*
Creamy Coleslaw*
Water with lemon

DAY 11

BREAKFAST

2 rashers back bacon or turkey bacon
½ grapefruit
1 slice toasted granary bread
Hot water with juice of ½ lemon, or herbal tea

LUNCH

175 g (6 oz) poached, barbecued or grilled salmon topped with
    Celebration Salsa*
Simple Greens and Garlic*
Water with lemon

SNACK

4–6 carrot and celery sticks with Cucumber and Yoghurt Dressing* for
    dipping

DINNER

115 g (4 oz) ground buffalo or lean sirloin meat patty
Swede and Nutmeg*
Broccoli or Asparagus with Sesame Seeds*
Water with lemon

DAY 12

BREAKFAST

150 g (5½ oz) natural low-fat yoghurt, mixed with 70 g (2½ oz) chopped apple or berries and 2 tablespoons ground or milled flaxseed. Add ¼ teaspoon raw honey and/or cinnamon or nutmeg to taste if desired.

1 egg, boiled, poached or scrambled; garnish with fresh salsa if desired.

Hot water with juice of ½ lemon, or herbal tea

LUNCH

Tossed Turkey and Spinach Salad*

1 medium orange

Water with lemon

SNACK

35 g (1¼ oz) almonds or 70 g (2½ oz) pumpkin seeds

DINNER

Garlic Chickpeas and Pasta*

55–115 g (2–9 oz) sliced cucumber, carrots and radishes with Cucumber and Yoghurt Dressing*

Water with lemon

DAY 13

BREAKFAST
1 poached or boiled egg
Banana in Bark*
Hot water with juice of ½ lemon, or herbal tea

LUNCH
Tuna Melt*
1 medium apple or pear
Water with lemon

SNACK
115 g (4 oz) low-fat cottage cheese, mixed with mandarin orange
    slices and 2 tablespoons flaxseed

DINNER
Colourful Turkey Casserole*
Beetroot and Orange Salad*
1 slice toasted granary bread
Water with lemon

DAY 14

BREAKFAST
Flaxseed and Fruit Smoothie*
150 g (5 oz) poached or grilled salmon
Hot water with juice of ½ lemon, or herbal tea

LUNCH
Turkey, Apple and Spinach Pitta*
Carrot and Orange Salad*
Water with lemon

SNACK
1 medium orange or 2 tangerines

DINNER
Lemon Hot Fish*
Asian Cabbage*
75 g (2¾ oz) couscous
Water with lemon

DAY 15

BREAKFAST
Favourite Feta Frittata*
125 ml (4 fl oz) orange or grapefruit juice
Hot water with juice of ½ lemon, or herbal tea

LUNCH
Orange-Ginger Salmon*
Creamy Coleslaw*
Water with lemon

SNACK
140 g (5 oz) of berries, tossed with 1 tablespoon natural low-fat
    yoghurt and 2 tablespoons flaxseed

DINNER
Spicy Kale and Beans*
100 g (3½ oz) brown rice; may cook in organic chicken, beef or
    vegetable broth for flavour
Water with lemon

DAY 16

BREAKFAST

70 g (2½ oz) whole-grain or bran cereal with 2 tablespoons ground or
milled flaxseed, 140 g (5 oz) fresh berries and 225 ml (8 fl oz)
skimmed milk

1 turkey sausage

Hot water with juice of ½ lemon, or herbal tea

LUNCH

175 g (6 oz) barbecued chicken or turkey breast

Sauerkraut Salad*

1 sliced tomato with salt, pepper, dried Italian seasoning and olive oil

Water with lemon

SNACK

1 medium apple or pear

DINNER

Fish New Orleans Style*

Beetroots and Brussels Sprouts*

100 g (3½ oz) brown rice; may cook in organic chicken, beef or
vegetable broth for flavour

Water with lemon

DAY 17

BREAKFAST
1 boiled or poached egg
1 medium orange
35 g (1¼ oz) almonds
Hot water with juice of ½ lemon, or herbal tea

LUNCH
140–175 g (5–6 oz) grilled or poached salmon
Cucumber and Yoghurt Dressing* as a condiment for the salmon
70 g (2½ oz) steamed asparagus
1 slice toasted granary bread
Water with lemon

SNACK
Banana in Bark*

DINNER
Garlic Chickpeas and Pasta*
50 g (1¾ oz) spinach salad
Water with lemon

DAY 18

BREAKFAST
150 g (5½ oz) natural low-fat yoghurt, mixed with 70 g (2½ oz)
    chopped apple or berries and 2 tablespoons ground or milled
    flaxseed. Add ½ teaspoon of raw honey and/or cinnamon or nut-
    meg to taste if desired.
2 rashers turkey bacon
Hot water with juice of ½ lemon, or herbal tea

LUNCH
175 g (6 oz) black beans and 100 g (3½ oz) brown rice
Marinated Cucumber, Radish and Onion Salad*
1 wholemeal tortilla
Water with lemon

SNACK
4–6 celery and carrot sticks
Ginger-Lime Dressing*

DINNER
Cauliflower Crab Cakes*
Broccoli or Asparagus with Sesame Seeds*
100 g (3½ oz) brown rice; may cook in organic chicken, beef or
    vegetable broth for flavour
Water with lemon

DAY 19

BREAKFAST
Asparagus Omelette*
2 rashers turkey bacon
125 ml (4 fl oz) grapefruit or orange juice
Hot water with juice of ½ lemon, or herbal tea

LUNCH
Favourite Chicken Salad* on bed of fresh spinach
Carrot and Orange Salad*
Water with lemon

SNACK
140 g (5 oz) of berries, tossed with 1 tablespoon natural low-fat
    yoghurt and 2 tablespoons flaxseed

DINNER
Nest of Beans and Greens*
Simple Cheese on Toast*
Water with lemon

DAY 20

BREAKFAST

70 g (2½ oz) whole-grain or bran cereal, with 2 tablespoons ground or
 milled flaxseed, 70 g (2½ oz) fresh berries and 225 ml (8 fl oz)
 skimmed milk
1 boiled egg
Hot water with juice of ½ lemon, or herbal tea

LUNCH

Open-Faced Veggie Cheeseburger*
Marinated Cucumber, Radish and Onion Salad*
Water with lemon

SNACK

1 medium orange or 2 tangerines

DINNER

Baked Fish with Basil*
Broccoli and Cauliflower in Lime Dressing*
75 g (2½ oz) cooked carrots; may season with dill, Italian seasoning or
 a butter substitute if desired.
Water with lemon

DAY 21

BREAKFAST
1 poached egg
½ grapefruit
1 slice toasted granary bread
Hot water with juice of ½ lemon, or herbal tea

LUNCH
Turkey and Asparagus Wrap*
1 medium apple or pear
Water with lemon

PARTY!
Celebration! In three weeks, you've probably lost 7–10 pounds (3–4.5 kilograms). Instead of having your everyday snack, have a party. Invite your friends over and let them in on your secret. Serve the following:

Marinated vegetable potpourri

Simple Cheese on Toast*

Spinach dip and raw vegetables

Sparkling water with a splash of cranberry or orange juice served in champagne glasses; drop in a few raspberries for colour and zing. (Make sure the cranberry juice is 100% fruit juice and not the kind that is sweetened with high-fructose corn syrup.)

DINNER
175 g (6 oz) Salmon with Dill and Lemon*
20 g (¾ oz) spinach salad
100 g (3½ oz) brown rice; may cook in organic chicken, beef or vegetable broth for flavour
Water with lemon

DAY 22

BREAKFAST
1 egg, scrambled in olive oil. Sprinkle liberally with dill or dried Italian
   seasoning if desired.
1 slice toasted granary bread; spread with a butter substitute if desired.
1 small orange
Hot water with juice of ½ lemon, or herbal tea

LUNCH
Savoury Spinach and Salmon Salad*
Cabbage-Apple Salad*
Water with lemon

SNACK
1 medium orange or 2 tangerines

DINNER
Baked Fish with Basil*
Broccoli or Asparagus with Sesame Seeds*
Mashed Cauliflower*
Water with lemon

DAY 23

BREAKFAST
70 g (2½ oz) whole-grain or bran cereal with 2 tablespoons ground or
     milled flaxseed, 70 g (2½ oz) berries and 225 g (8 fl oz) skimmed
     milk
1 boiled egg
Hot water with juice of ½ lemon, or herbal tea

LUNCH
175 g (6 oz) sliced turkey or chicken breast
Spinach Salad with Beetroot in Cottage Cheese*
Water with lemon

SNACK
35 g (1¼ oz) almonds or 70 g (2½ oz) pumpkin seeds

DINNER
Spicy Kale and Beans*
1 medium apple or pear
1 slice granary bread
Water with lemon

DAY 24

BREAKFAST
115–175 g (4–6 oz) grilled or poached salmon
Yoghurt and Fruit Parfait*
Hot water with juice of ½ lemon, or herbal tea

LUNCH
Veggie Burger*
Best Baked Beans*
Cabbage-Apple Salad*
Water with lemon

SNACK
4–6 celery and carrot sticks
Ginger-Lime Dressing* for dipping

DINNER
Rosemary-Baked Chicken Breast*
Green and Yellow Veggie Hash*
100 g (3½ oz) cooked brown rice
Water with lemon

DAY 25

BREAKFAST
Asparagus Omelette*
2 rashers turkey bacon
175 g (6 fl oz) grapefruit or orange juice
Hot water with juice of ½ lemon, or herbal tea

LUNCH
Not Your Ordinary Tuna Salad*
Water with lemon
Swede and Nutmeg*

SNACK
Banana in Bark*

DINNER
Grilled 115 g (4 oz) fillet of lean beef
Cruciferous Couscous*
Roasted Beetroot*
Water with lemon

DAY 26

BREAKFAST

1 poached egg

½ grapefruit

1 slice toasted granary bread; spread with 1 teaspoon of all fruit jam or butter substitute if desired.

Hot water with juice of ½ lemon, or herbal tea

LUNCH

1 turkey hot dog, grilled

Kale and Sauerkraut*

1 sliced tomato; drizzle with olive oil and balsamic vinegar if desired.

Water with lemon

SNACK

115 g (4 oz) low-fat cottage cheese, mixed with mandarin orange slices and 2 tablespoons ground or milled flaxseed

DINNER

Fish with Citrus Marinade*

Simple Greens and Garlic*

Spinach and Feta Brown Rice*

Water with lemon

DAY 27

BREAKFAST

150 g (5½ oz) natural low-fat yoghurt, mixed with 35 g (1¼ oz)
    chopped apple and 2 tablespoons ground or milled flaxseed. Add ¼
    teaspoon of raw honey and/or cinnamon or nutmeg to taste if
    desired.

2 rashers turkey bacon

Hot water with juice of ½ lemon, or herbal tea

LUNCH

Cauliflower and Turkey Bacon Soup*

Simple Cheese on Toast*

Water with lemon

SNACK

35 g (1¼ oz) almonds or 70 g (2½ oz) pumpkin seeds

DINNER

175 g (6 oz) grilled fish (drizzle with lemon or marinate with lemon
    juice or salsa)

Lemon-Curry Cauliflower and Kale*

75 g (2¾ oz) steamed carrots seasoned with salt, pepper and dried dill
    if desired.

Water with lemon

DAY 28

BREAKFAST
70 g (2½ oz) whole-grain or bran cereal, with 2 tablespoons ground or
    milled flaxseed, 70 g (2½ oz) fresh berries and 225 ml (8 fl oz)
    skimmed milk
1 boiled egg
Hot water with juice of ½ lemon, or herbal tea

LUNCH
Favourite Chicken Salad*
Beetroot and Orange Salad*
Water with lemon

SNACK
1 medium orange or 2 tangerines

DINNER
Baked Fish with Basil*
Dressed-Up Asparagus*
100 g (3½ oz) brown rice; may cook in organic chicken, beef or vege-
    table broth for flavour
Water with lemon

DAY 29

BREAKFAST

2 rashers turkey bacon

1 slice toasted granary bread; spread with 1 teaspoon all fruit jam or
butter substitute if desired.

½ grapefruit

Hot water with juice of ½ lemon, or herbal tea

LUNCH

Spicy Kale and Beans*

1 small sliced cucumber and 1 sliced tomato; may dress with low-fat
balsamic vinegar dressing

Water with lemon

SNACK

35 g (1¼ oz) almonds or 70 g (2½ oz) pumpkin seeds

DINNER

Lemon Hot Fish*

75 g (2¾ oz) steamed broccoli tossed with olive oil and garlic

30 g (1 oz) wholemeal pasta, mixed with diced tomato, olive oil and
fresh basil

Water with lemon

DAY 30

BREAKFAST
Flaxseed and Fruit Smoothie*
115–175 g (4–6 oz) poached or grilled salmon
Hot water with juice of ½ lemon, or herbal tea

LUNCH
Veggie Burger* patty (no bun)
Sauerkraut Salad*
Sliced apple
Water with lemon

SNACK
150 g (5½ oz) natural low-fat yoghurt, mixed with 1 tablespoon orange
    juice concentrate, 1 medium orange and 2 tablespoons ground or
    milled flaxseed

DINNER
175 g (6 oz) baked, grilled or barbecued chicken breast
Indian-Style Brussels Sprouts*
90 g (3¼ oz) steamed courgette
1 slice toasted granary bread; spread with 1 teaspoon butter substitute
    if desired.
Water with lemon

Sticking to this nutritional plan will go a long way towards
balancing your hormones and will help you lose weight;
however, for those wanting to get rid of oestrogen dominance
and belly fat quickly and for good, there are two more important steps you have to take. The next two chapters will tell
you exactly what they are.

STEP 2:
USE PROGESTERONE:
THE SIMPLE WAY TO A FLAT
BELLY

(4)

Although the title of this chapter might sound too good to be true, the success of thousands of patients has shown this to be a reality. By boosting your body's progesterone levels, you can take an important step towards correcting your underlying condition of oestrogen dominance and finally lose those pounds. You will also make a large stride in improving your overall health and well being.

how to safely and effectively boost declining progesterone levels

If your progesterone production has declined and you are oestrogen dominant, then common sense would indicate that in order to reestablish hormonal equilibrium, you have to add progesterone back into your body. The theory is very simple, but unfortunately there is a great deal of confusion about hormone replacement therapies.

Over the last several years, hormone replacement has frequently been in the news. In magazine articles and on television, celebrities have bandied around terms like *natural, bio-identical, synthetic* and *pharmaceutical* as if they were interchangeable. They are not.

Natural human hormones are produced within your body by the ovaries or testes, the adrenal glands and the hypothalamus. These hormones travel through the bloodstream to fit into specific hormone receptor sites located throughout your body and brain. Each hormone receptor site will recognise the specific molecular structure of only a single type of hormone. This means that a receptor site for progesterone will not recognise oestrogen or testosterone; it will recognise only the molecular structure of progesterone.

Natural human hormones attach to their receptor sites like keys fitting into locks. The chemical term for this key-and-lock phenomenon is *relative binding affinity* (RBA). Natural human hormones have a 100 per cent RBA for their respective receptor sites.

what every woman needs to know: the danger of synthetic hormones

Bio-identical hormones are derived from plants, usually soybeans or wild yams. This biochemical process ensures that the molecular structure of bio-identical hormones is identical to that of the natural human hormones produced in the body. When introduced into the body, bio-identical hormones *fit perfectly* into the hormone receptor lock and trigger exactly the same response as the one previously fostered by the hormones produced in the ovaries or testes, the adrenal gland and the hypothalamus.

Bio-identical hormones also have a 100 per cent RBA for the hormone receptor sites within the body. Because the body recognises and accepts bio-identical hormones just as it would recognise and accept naturally occurring human hormones, bio-identical hormone replacement is both safe and effective.

The molecular structure of natural human hormones cannot be patented; thus, neither can the identical molecular structure of bio-identical hormones. Without a patent, how could pharmaceutical companies protect their formulations and, most important, their profits? The answer is that they can't. Consequently, for almost three-quarters of a century, pharmaceutical companies have been developing, patenting and marketing hormones that have a slightly different molecular structure from natural human hormones and bio-identical hormones. The pharmaceutically produced and patented hormones are correctly referred to as synthetic hormones. The list of synthetic hormones on the market today includes such brand names as Premarin, Preminque and Kliovance. There are many others.

Synthetic hormones have shapes that are not found in nature. They fit poorly with the body's hormone receptors and therefore produce unnatural chemical reactions and striking alterations in biological activity. Their RBA is often much less than 100 per cent, which results in side effects and health risks. Premarin, for instance, is metabolised horse oestrogen with a low affinity for binding with any human hormone receptor. Premarin is also 49.3 per cent oestrone

(E1), the cancer-promoting oestrogen. This is almost ten times the percentage that occurs naturally within the body.

Many medical studies have substantiated the dangers of synthetic hormone replacement. In July 2002, the National Institutes of Health (NIH) in the United States halted a large study examining the effects of a widely used synthetic hormone, Prempro, which combines the altered molecular structures for both oestrogen and progesterone. The study, which was one of five major studies in a large clinical trial called the Women's Health Initiative, was discontinued because the synthetic hormones were found to increase a woman's risk of breast cancer as well as heart disease, blood clots and stroke. Later findings also linked synthetic hormone replacement to an increased risk for Alzheimer's disease. The findings were published in *The Journal of the American Medical Association*.

Unfortunately, bio-identical progesterone is often confused with synthetically produced progestin. The Women's Health Initiative used progestin, *not* bio-identical progesterone. There is no documented evidence in the scientific literature of any cases of cancer resulting from treatment with bio-identical progesterone.

In contrast, studies reported in both the International Society for Preventive Oncology's *Cancer Detection and Prevention Journal* (1999) and the International Union Against Cancer's *International Cancer Journal* (2005) found that women who used synthetic progestins plus oestrogen had a significantly higher risk of breast cancer, whereas women using bio-identical progesterone plus synthetic oestrogens had a lower risk of breast cancer than women using oestrogen alone.

marketing a dangerous lie

If bio-identical hormone replacement is so safe, you might be wondering why so many physicians continue to prescribe synthetic hormones. The answer is a combination of ignorance, confusion and marketing. Pharmaceutical companies make billions selling synthetic hormone products. In terms of the safety of synthetic versus bio-identical hormone replacement, pharmaceutical companies have a lot to lose. Consequently, these companies spend millions marketing synthetic hormones to physicians by sponsoring continuing medical education (CME) programmes, office lunch presentations and off-site forums at resort locations.

In her book, *The Truth About the Drug Companies*, Dr Marcia Angell, former editor in chief of *The New England Journal of Medicine*, states: 'Drug companies have become vast marketing machines wielding nearly limitless influence over medical research, education and how doctors do their jobs.'

There are volumes of solid, credible clinical trials and medical studies that validate the safety and efficacy of bio-identical hormone therapies. Unfortunately, the medical research institutions and universities that publish these studies do not have the budget to hire a sales force to go out into the field to educate physicians. Consequently, most doctors continue to remain unenlightened regarding the science behind the safe treatment option of bio-identical hormones.

how bio-identical progesterone kick-starts weight loss at a cellular level

Bio-identical progesterone neutralises oestrogen dominance, thereby kick-starting weight loss at a cellular level. Here's what happens.

First, progesterone eliminates the hypothyroid condition. Oestrogen causes food calories to be stored as fat; the thyroid hormone causes fat calories to be turned into usable energy. Oestrogen and the thyroid hormone therefore have opposing actions. Oestrogen dominance inhibits thyroid action and lowers the rate of metabolism of the body. Progesterone inhibits oestrogen action, thereby allowing the thyroid hormone to function properly. In other words, progesterone triggers a metabolic response that allows weight loss to occur.

Second, when progesterone is added back into the body, it acts as a natural diuretic, which helps to reduce bloating.

Finally, when progesterone and oestrogen levels are re-balanced, the rapid release of insulin is tempered. The result is normalised blood sugar levels and reduced food cravings.

the health benefits of bio-identical progesterone

In addition to helping with weight loss, bio-identical progesterone brings numerous health benefits.

protection from cancer

As previously described, oestrogen increases cell growth, and when unchecked, this cell growth can result in cancer. In

contrast, bio-identical progesterone replacement can neu-
tralise or reduce oestrogen's ability to stimulate cell growth.
According to several medical studies, when internal progesterone levels are boosted to balance oestrogen levels, there is
not enough extra oestrogen circulating within the body to
stimulate oestrogen receptor-positive tumour growth.

Dr Uzzi Reiss, founder of the Beverly Hills Anti-Aging
Center and co-author of *Natural Hormone Balance for Women*,
explains as follows:

> *Progesterone is the most protective breast hormone. At an*
> *infertility clinic at Johns Hopkins, Linda Cowan published a*
> *study in the early 1980s. She followed two groups of women*
> *for more than 20 years. There aren't many studies like this.*
> *What's unique about these women is that one group had*
> *blocked fallopian tubes, and the other group had progesterone*
> *deficiency. The only long-term health effect the women with*
> *blocked tubes had was the inability to get pregnant. But more*
> *than 20 years later, the group with progesterone deficiency had*
> *tenfold more cancer.*

How could this be? It's very simple: progesterone functions
to inhibit cells from replicating. Progesterone increases the
activity of a gene called P53, which protects us from cancer. It
also down-regulates and decreases the function of BCL2, a
gene that is a marker for cancer.

The role of hormone balance in the development and prevention of hormone-dependent cancers is still a subject of
much controversy in the conventional medical community.
More research is definitely needed in this area; however, in

more than a decade of treating thousands of women suffering from hormone imbalances, I have only had two patients who were later diagnosed with breast cancer. This is far below the national average. Breast cancer is now the most common cancer in the UK. Research in 2005 showed that more than 45,500 women were diagnosed with breast cancer, which is about 125 women a day. Eight or 10 breast cancers are diagnosed in women aged 50 and over. In the last 10 years, breast cancer rates in the UK have increased by 13 per cent. Wouldn't it be nice if someday we would read about a scientific study that tracked a huge reduction in breast cancer rates because every woman in Britain augmented her body's progesterone level as soon as her hormone levels began to shift?

cardiac health

Bio-identical progesterone replacement is also good for heart health. Because heart disease is the number one killer of women in the industrialised world (over 60,000 women die of heart disease in the UK each year), the effect of progesterone on cardiac health has been an area of extensive research. You will recall that the Women's Health Initiative trial indicated that synthetic oestrogen plus progestin increased cardiac risk. The good news is that researchers have proven that a hormone replacement regime consisting of both bio-identical oestrogen and bio-identical progesterone serves to reduce coronary vascular activity. In other words, whether progesterone is produced within the body naturally or is a bio-identical formulation added back into the body, it definitively balances oestrogen and has a cardioprotective effect.

osteoporosis prevention

Progesterone is also responsible for the stimulation of bone building that can prevent or treat osteoporosis. Dr Morris Noteloviz, author of *Estrogen, Yes or No?* states, 'Progesterone receptors are present in osteoblasts. Based on *in vivo* (in the body) and clinical studies, it is now believed that bio-identical progesterone replacement may stimulate new bone formation, although the mechanism has not yet been identified.'

A 1996 study published in *The Journal of the American Medical Association* found that women using bio-identical progesterone cream experienced an average of 7 to 8 per cent bone mineral density increase in the first year, 4 to 5 per cent in the second year and 3 to 4 per cent in the third year. Untreated women in this category typically lose 1.5 per cent bone mineral density per year. For the treatment and prevention of bone density loss, no other form of hormone replacement or dietary supplementation has had as high a level of positive response as bio-identical progesterone.

PMT relief

Have you or anyone you know ever suffered from premenstrual tension (PMT)? If so, here is more good news about progesterone. In the early 1950s, a theory was advanced within the medical community that PMT was caused by unopposed oestrogen during the luteal phase of your menstrual cycle. The luteal phase is the time period beginning with the day after ovulation and running through the remainder of your menstrual cycle (it ends the day before your next period). Typically, the duration of the luteal phase lasts between ten and sixteen days, and is generally consistent from cycle to cycle, averaging for most women at fourteen days. To test this theory, researchers administered bio-identical progesterone by intramuscular injection, vaginal or rectal suppository or subcutaneous pellets. Bio-identical progesterone resolved PMS symptoms in 83 per cent of the women in the study.

improved memory and moods

Oestrogen and progesterone must be in balance for the brain to function properly. Oestrogen increases brain stimulation and fosters clear thinking and good memory. Progesterone is very important to the central nervous system; it has been proven to promote healthy sleep patterns and a sense of calm. Progesterone is often referred to as the 'feel-good' hormone. Although progesterone's effect on mood and sense of well being is very relevant, there is also new evidence that it might play an even more critical role in long-term mental functioning. Recent research has shown that an imbalance in oestrogen and progesterone levels could be a precursor to Alzheimer's disease.

improved quality of life

Medical research studies provide clear physiological and biochemical evidence of the many health benefits of bio-identical progesterone replacement. For instance, the Mayo Clinic published a study in the *Journal of Women's Health* in

2000 that showed that women who included bio-identical progesterone in their hormone replacement regime were more satisfied with their overall quality of life. The study participants also reported that they felt an improvement in several other health areas, including relief of sleep disturbances, hot flushes, anxiety and symptoms of depression.

forms of bio-identical progesterone

Bio-identical progesterone can be administered as a cream, a pill, a capsule, a gelcap, drops under the tongue or a suppository. Fortunately, for those who don't like taking pills, topical creams have been shown to be the most effective way of administering bio-identical progesterone. If you take bio-identical progesterone in a pill, it must first go through the liver to be metabolised. Some of the active substance is automatically excreted in the faeces. The remaining progesterone must be metabolised into more than thirty-five biochemical substances before it can enter the bloodstream. This means that only a fraction of the progesterone contained in the pill makes its way into your bloodstream. When applied to your skin, however, the progesterone goes directly into your bloodstream. Once it is in your bloodstream, all of the progesterone in the cream travels to the progesterone receptor sites and is utilised by progesterone target tissues. Very simply, bio-identical progesterone cream allows the body to recognise and use the bio-identical hormone replacement in exactly the same way it would use progesterone produced by the ovaries. Furthermore, the body's response to the cream is more immediate with a lower dosage.

HOW TO USE PROGESTERONE ON THE PLAN

To use bio-identical progesterone, follow these guidelines:

- If you're a woman who is still menstruating regularly, apply the cream twice daily from days 8 to 26 of your cycle. In other words, *do not apply when menstruating*.
- If you're a woman who is no longer menstruating due to the menopause or a hysterectomy, who is peri-menopausal or who is having irregular periods, apply the cream twice daily for twenty-five days. Then take five days off. (You may begin using the cream on any day you choose.)
- If you're a woman who is also on a regime of bio-identical oestrogen, you should apply bio-identical progesterone cream twice daily, every day. (Bio-identical oestrogen replacement will be discussed later.)
- If you're a man older than forty, you should also apply the cream twice daily for twenty-five days. Then take five days off. (You may begin using the cream on any day you choose.)

Bio-identical progesterone cream is readily available without a prescription in the US. You can purchase formulations at compounding pharmacies with a physician's prescription or over the counter at most health food stores and some natural product websites. However, over-the-counter bio-identical progesterone cream is not available in the UK: it is only available via private prescription.

I stumbled onto the discrepancy ten years ago when I first began treating patients. Determining from their symptoms that my patients needed bio-identical progesterone replacement, I would recommend that they purchase an over-the-counter progesterone cream and apply it twice a day, yet I didn't direct them to any specific brand. I would then ask them to return in six weeks so I could monitor their response and symptom improvement.

After six weeks, some patients reported great improvement – or even elimination of – their symptoms. Others reported less than satisfying results. The discrepancy led me to think that certain products were more helpful than others. Drawing on my pharmacological background, I did some research to determine which formulations work the best and why.

what to look for in a progesterone cream

The ideal progesterone cream is a bio-identical formulation of progesterone and not just a mixture of natural remedies for hormone replacement. The confusion between the two is caused by the fact that the parent molecule for progesterone comes from a substance known as diosgenin, which is found in soya and in Mexican wild yam. Many products on the market today that contain soya or Mexican wild yam claim to be natural progesterone; however, they won't work in the body in the same way that bio-identical progesterone does. Until the diosgenin molecule is converted in a laboratory from its original molecular structure to that of bio-identical progesterone, the body will not recognise it. Consequently, soya or Mexican wild yam in a raw state will not effectively impact the underlying hormonal imbalance or its symptoms.

For the best and purest product on the market, the bio-identical progesterone used in the cream must meet the US Pharmacopoeia gold standard for quality. This should be clearly marked on the product label.

In addition, the lab in which the bio-identical progesterone is compounded should operate under the strict guidelines of the National Association of Compounding Pharmacists. This is not required by law, so not all product manufacturers go to the trouble or expense.

The progesterone molecule in the cream should be designed to be released over time. This is critical, because if the cream is immediately absorbed through the skin, it will result in a quick spike in progesterone levels and a temporary rather than constant relief of symptoms. The importance of a time-controlled delivery system is that optimal hormonal balance is restored continuously so that users of the cream experience continuous relief of their symptoms throughout the day. The term *liposomal formulation* or *liposomal delivery* should be clearly visible on the product label.

You can find information about my personal formulation of bio-identical progesterone cream on my website www.hormonewell.com.

Prior to his death in 2003, Dr John R Lee, the primary author of the *What Your Doctor May Not Tell You About Menopause* series and a recognised pioneer in the field of bio-identical hormone replacement, worked with co-author Virginia Hopkins to provide a list of reviewed and approved over-the-counter progesterone creams. You can find his original listing in the back of his books. Today, Ms Hopkins continues Dr Lee's mission by regularly updating his original list of preferred creams on his website (www.johnleemd.com/store/resource_progesterone.html).

Remember oestrogen-dominant Evelyn and Richard from Chapter 2? Although they were both sceptical that simply rubbing on a cream twice a day would have any real benefit, they agreed to give it a try. Just six weeks later Evelyn called to report the following:

> *Dr Randolph, I honestly didn't hold much stock in what you told me, but because I felt desperate, I was willing to give any-thing a try. Within three weeks of using your progesterone cream, my stomach felt less bloated, and I weighed 6 pounds less. I also found that I felt calmer throughout the day, and at night I slept without waking for the first time in years.*
>
> *Richard has actually lost 8 pounds in just six weeks. Soon after he started using your cream, he began to act more like his old self. He started coming home, and instead of plopping down on the sofa with a beer, he would take a thirty- to forty-minute walk. He has also begun to have more energy in our bedroom, if you know what I mean. We both feel like your pro-gesterone cream is a miracle potion.*

Bio-identical progesterone replacement is no miracle potion, but when you restore the hormone that your body is missing, the results will often feel miraculous. Because boosting your deficient progesterone level is a critical first step in neutralis-ing an underlying condition of oestrogen dominance, don't wait until you've finished this book to get started. The sooner you begin using bio-identical progesterone cream, the better chance you have of making quick progress towards your weight-loss and waist-size goals.

STEP 3:
TAKE THE RIGHT SUPPLEMENTS
TO SUPPORT, NOT SABOTAGE,
YOUR HORMONE BALANCE

Over the last several years, I have researched and tested hordes of nutritional supplements. My goal has been to identify those supplements that could positively influence oestrogen metabolism. I have found a select group of supplements that will enhance healthy hormone balance and thus promote weight loss and weight management. These are described below.

Calcium D-Glucarate

Calcium D-glucarate is a natural substance that promotes the body's detoxification process and supports hormonal balance. Calcium D-glucarate facilitates the detoxification process by inhibiting the reabsorption of oestrogen-like toxins into the bloodstream, allowing them to leave the body and be excreted in the faeces.

Calcium D-glucarate has been found to lower unhealthy oestrogen levels in animals and thereby inhibit the development or progression of cancer.

✓ TAKE 1,000 MG OF CALCIUM D-GLUCARATE TWICE DAILY.

Diindolylmethane (DIM)

Diindolylmethane (DIM) is a phytonutrient akin to the indole-3-carbinol (I3C) found in cruciferous vegetables. DIM has unique hormonal benefits. It supports the activity of enzymes that improve oestrogen metabolism by increasing the levels of 2-hydroxyestrone – that is, the good oestrogen. When taken as part of a healthy diet, DIM helps to relieve PMT symptoms and to promote fat loss and healthy oestrogen metabolism.

In men, DIM also promotes its own metabolism. This means that it allows for greater testosterone activity. Men who take DIM supplements will benefit biochemically because DIM promotes an optimal testosterone-to-oestrogen ratio.

✓ WOMEN SHOULD TAKE 200 MG OF DIM PER DAY; MEN SHOULD TAKE 400 MG PER DAY.

The B Vitamins

The B vitamins – B_1, B_2, B_3, B_5, B_6, B_{12} and folate – do a lot within your body to support oestrogen detoxification.

Conversely, if your body is deficient in B vitamins, you will have higher levels of circulating oestrogen. By now, you definitely know that increased oestrogen levels lead to oestrogen dominance – and oestrogen dominance will most certainly lead to weight gain and the inability to get rid of that weight.

B vitamins also impact oestrogen activity for the hormone receptors at the cellular level. Clinical studies have shown that high levels of intracellular (i.e., within the cell) B_6 can decrease the binding response at the oestrogen hormone receptor site. What happens at the cellular level is sort of like an internal game of musical chairs: if the music stops and B_6 sits down in the 'oestrogen chair', then the oestrogen molecule is out of the game.

✓ BECAUSE THE B VITAMINS WORK TOGETHER TO PERFORM SUCH VITAL TASKS AT THE CELLULAR LEVEL, YOU SHOULD TAKE A B-COMPLEX VITAMIN, NOT JUST ONE OR TWO OF THE B VITAMINS. Take a B-complex that has 50–100 mg each of thiamine (B_1), riboflavin (B_2), niacin (B_3), pantothenic acid (B_5) and B_6 (a water-soluble vitamin that exists in three major chemical forms: pyridoxine, pyridoxal and pyridoxamine), along with PABA, choline, inositol, 50 micrograms (mcg) of B_{12} and 400 mcg of folic acid.

Vitamin E

Years ago, researchers studied the effects of vitamin E in reducing the difficulties of the menopause, and most of these studies found vitamin E to be helpful. Vitamin E has also been shown to reduce PMT-related breast tenderness, nervousness, depression, headache, fatigue and insomnia. Newer research suggests that low vitamin E levels are linked to oestrogen dominance. Furthermore, vitamin E deficiency has been found to inhibit oestrogen detoxification.

✓ TAKE 400 IU OF VITAMIN E PER DAY.

Calcium-Magnesium Combo

Most women and men find it difficult to get the recommended 1,200–1,500 mg of calcium per day from their diet. Calcium intake should therefore be supplemented with a calcium-magnesium combination supplement. The right kind of fat is necessary for calcium availability in the soft tissues and to promote calcium elevation in the bloodstream so that muscles contract properly and maintain their tone, nerves function smoothly, blood clots when needed and bones and teeth remain strong and healthy. Women who believe they are getting enough calcium through diet and supplements may be sabotaging themselves if they do not include enough of the right oils (i.e. extra-virgin olive, rapeseed or flaxseed oils) in their diets. Also, because this diet includes minimum animal products and sodium and little or no sugar or caffeine, your body should better retain its nutritional and supplemental calcium.

Magnesium is another element that helps the body to eliminate excess oestrogen. For women, magnesium levels tend to fall at certain times during the menstrual cycle. These shifts in magnesium levels can upset an optimal calcium-magnesium ratio. When the two minerals are in proper balance, the body better absorbs and assimilates the calcium it needs and also allows calcium to migrate from tissue and organs where it doesn't belong.

Without magnesium, calcium might not be fully utilised. Underabsorption of calcium can lead to menstrual cramps. As with a vitamin E deficiency, when the body does not have enough magnesium to support calcium absorption, many women report PMT symptoms such as mood swings, fatigue, headaches and sleeplessness.

Premenstrual chocolate craving is a phenomenon that has puzzled many physicians. They have been unable to explain why some women have this overwhelming urge to eat lots of chocolate right before their periods, yet at other times of the month the women's chocolate cravings are not as strong. The PMT-chocolate connection makes a lot of sense because chocolate is very high in magnesium.

Keeping a balance of calcium and magnesium is critical for optimal physical functioning and for hormone balance.

✓ YOU SHOULD TAKE A CALCIUM-MAGNESIUM SUPPLEMENT THAT CONTAINS A RATIO OF TWO PARTS CALCIUM (1,500 MG) TO ONE PART MAGNESIUM (750 MG).

7-Keto Dehydroepiandrosterone (DHEA)

Dehydroepiandrosterone (DHEA) is one of the hormones produced by the adrenal glands. After being secreted by the adrenal glands, DHEA circulates in the bloodstream as DHEA-sulfate (DHEAS) and is converted, as needed, into other hormones. Since it is a precursor to testosterone, DHEA may help to build muscle. It is very unusual for anyone under the age of thirty-five or forty to have low DHEA levels. As we age, however, the body's production of DHEA declines, so people older than forty can most definitely become DHEA-deficient.

Although many anti-ageing enthusiasts are familiar with DHEA, far fewer are likely to be aware of its metabolite, 7-keto DHEA, which within the body to safely boost immune function and help reduce body fat. The term *7-keto DHEA* is in fact a brand name for the chemical compound 3-acetyl-7-dehydroepiandrosterone. Human blood levels of both DHEA and 7-keto DHEA tend to rise and fall in a similar pattern with age: increasing until the twenties, beginning to decline in the thirties and continuing to decline until the levels are reduced by about 50 per cent by the age of fifty. Clinical studies have shown that as 7-keto DHEA levels go down in middle age, body weight tends to goes up.

Weight loss is stimulated by 7-keto DHEA through a process called *thermogenesis*, the creation of heat at a cellular level. The more thermogenesis, the higher the metabolic rate and the more that fat is literally burned up as energy. Studies have also demonstrated that 7-keto DHEA does not accumulate in the body over time and that it is free of unhealthy side effects.

Supplementation with 7-keto DHEA is significantly beneficial for increasing the rate at which the body converts stored fat into energy. Because 7-keto DHEA is a natural hormone metabolite, it benefits the body in two ways: it helps to restore hormone balance while also working internally to melt away those unwanted pounds.

✓ TAKE 100 MG OF 7-KETO DHEA PER DAY, ONE CAPSULE EVERY MORNING.

Chitosan

Chitosan, which is processed from the shells of crustaceans such as prawns, lobster and crab, acts as a super fibre. Its swelling action creates a sensation of feeling full, thereby serving to suppress the appetite. In addition, the super-fibre characteristics of chitosan foster a natural cleansing process that is vital to weight loss.

Chitosan is also able to absorb six to ten times its weight in fat and oils. It then converts the fat molecules into a form that the human body does not absorb. Because chitosan causes less fat to enter the body, the body has to turn to previously stored body fat to burn for energy. The net result is weight loss.

✓ TAKE 750 MG TO 1 GRAM (G) OF CHITOSAN THREE TIMES A DAY WITH MEALS.

KEEPING THAT *FLAT* BELLY FOR LIFE

Are you concerned about putting the three steps – diet, progesterone and supplements – into an easy framework that you can use every day? This section shows you how to integrate these steps into your daily life and how to make hormone-healthy choices that support your weight-loss goals.

A fear of rebound weight gain is common in people who follow this three-step plan and finally take off those extra pounds around their middle. The good news is that these fears almost always prove to be unfounded. Years go by and people on this plan delightedly maintain their desired weight and waistlines.

Why does this plan work for life when other diets have short bursts of weight loss followed by permanent rebound weight gain? Because it is much more than a diet; it is a positive, healthy life plan. Stress and poor lifestyle choices can sabotage your hormone balance and thus your long-term weight loss.

This section provides a simple framework you can put into action every day to keep your weight off for the long term. We tell you how to make hormone-healthy choices in four key areas that affect your hormones and your weight: managing stress, getting enough sleep, staying active and boosting your adrenal glands. Finally, we end with a series of delicious recipes that you can enjoy while achieving your weight-loss goals.

KEEPING WEIGHT OFF
IN THE REAL WORLD

⑥

ad diets come and go. Unfortunately, so do those unwanted pounds. Fortunately for you, this plan offers a safe and effective alternative to yo-yo dieting. As you follow the three-step plan and move from *belly fat* to *belly flat*, you will discover a lifetime approach to keeping your hormones balanced and your waistline trim. To keep you on track, here are some helpful hints and reminders:

- Keep your bio-identical progesterone cream and your supplements by your toothbrush so that incorporating them into your daily regime quickly becomes automatic.
- Make a list before food shopping, and always shop on a full stomach. If you shop when you're hungry, you're more likely to be tempted by high-fat or high-calorie foods.
- Eat three meals a day and *never* skip breakfast. If you don't eat breakfast, your metabolism is more likely to

slow down to compensate for not receiving any new calories. In addition, you'll be more likely to experience low energy and food cravings later in the day.

- Eat slowly. It takes twenty minutes for your stomach to signal your brain that it is full. Try putting your fork down between bites, and have a drink of water to help you slow down.

- Do not eat in front of the television; when your attention is elsewhere, you're more likely to overeat.

- Avoid fast food, but when you have no other choice, order a grilled chicken 'sandwich' without the bun or mayonnaise. Most fast-food chains now also offer some type of side salad or fruit. Don't eat the dressing. Sprinkle with lemon juice instead.

- When eating out, avoid croutons and order low-fat salad dressing on the side; drizzle sparingly.

- Also when eating out, ask for a double order of broccoli or asparagus and dress with lemon juice to substitute for a buttery potato or rice dish.

- Keep a large bowl of broccoli and cauliflower florets ready for cooking or snacking.

- Although the sample daily menus include only one afternoon snack, if you get hungry between breakfast and lunch, eat another recommended snack.

- Try to eat dinner before 7 PM, and then do not eat again until breakfast. Drink water with lemon until bedtime.

- Keep small sandwich bags of chopped carrots and celery and nuts in the refrigerator. Grab them for a quick snack when you are on the run.

- Keep a weekly weight-loss journal and diet diary (see Appendix A). Record your weight, symptoms of hormone imbalance, stress level and exercise patterns. Measure your waistline circumference once a month.

Remember that the choices you make every minute of every day either work for you or against you. Unfortunately, people unknowingly sabotage their weight-loss efforts. There are four hidden saboteurs that can impact your weight: stress, lack of sleep, physical inactivity and insufficient supplementation.

stress and your hormones

Although too much oestrogen is the primary culprit that causes you to pack on those pounds, stress impacts the production of five other hormones that can influence your metabolism, your appetite and your food cravings. Three of the five hormones are produced by the walnut-sized adrenal glands located on top of each kidney. They are adrenalin, cortisol and dehydroepiandrosterone (DHEA). The other two hormones are ghrelin and leptin, which are produced by a small area in the middle of the brain called the hypothalamus. If stress has disrupted the balance of one or more of these five hormones, you will tend to always be hungry and will never feel full no matter how much you eat. The result is more fat stored around your middle.

According to Tene T Lewis, a health psychologist and lead researcher at Rush University Medical Center in Chicago, the pressures of a busy life can stimulate some bodies to conserve more fat. Dr Lewis's team of researchers found that the more stressors that were reported, the more weight that was gained over four years. This weight gain was not attributable to other variables like diet or exercise.

What are life stressors? The list of stressors typically cited by patients include the following: daily time-management issues, juggling work and family, being made redundant or fired, experiencing major money worries, losing a parent, going through a divorce and dealing with difficult infants, angry teenagers or ageing parents. Can you identify with these?

How does stress impact hormone levels? When the brain perceives some form of danger, it signals the adrenal glands to pump out more adrenalin, often referred to as the 'fight-or-flight' hormone. The sudden surge in adrenalin levels signals fat cells to quickly release energy. This energy rush stimulates flight. Once the body is out of danger, the brain continues to signal the adrenal glands that there is a temporary need to keep the adrenalin level elevated. Higher than normal adrenalin levels cause an increase in appetite, which encourages the body to eat more calories and replenish fat stores. In acute (short-term) stress situations, the adrenalin level will soon return to normal once the immediate appetite has been satisfied.

This brain-body hormone-stimulating phenomenon served human beings very well in times when people needed to avoid immediate dangers like being eaten by wolves or killed by invading armies. Today, however, the modern person in the United Kingdom is not frequently subjected to such immediate dangers.

Contemporary stressors, like worrying about paying the mortgage, doing the jobs of three people, dealing with an unhappy marriage or grappling with ongoing parenting issues, tend to be more long-term. A life stressor can be considered chronic if it persists for three or more months. Instead of pumping out more adrenalin, the adrenal glands respond to chronic stress by secreting more cortisol. Because chronic stress is ongoing, high cortisol levels do not subside until the stress is removed or the adrenal glands exhausted.

Over time, elevated cortisol levels can wreak havoc on your body. Sustained high cortisol levels destroy healthy muscle and bone, slow down healing and normal cell regeneration, deplete the necessary biochemicals to make other vital hormones, impair digestion, dull mental processes, interfere with healthy endocrine function and weaken the immune system. If you are stressed out, high cortisol levels will also compromise your metabolism and cement more pounds around your middle.

In addition, when the adrenals are chronically overworked and are straining to maintain high cortisol levels, they lose the capacity to produce DHEA in sufficient amounts. DHEA is necessary to moderate the balance of hormones in your body. When DHEA is produced at optimal levels, it functions to promote the loss of body fat. Double-blind clinical trials have found 100 mg per day of DHEA to be effective in decreasing body fat in older men. Conversely, when the body's DHEA levels are insufficient, body fat is more difficult to budge.

Recently, a female patient named Shirley complained that she had gained 15 pounds (7 kilograms) in the last nine months. She said she wouldn't be unhappy if she could only spread some of those pounds around to her 'stick-skinny legs' or to her arms or chest. The problem was that all 15 pounds had attached themselves to her middle.

Shirley reported that in the last eighteen months she had purchased a new home, moved across town and away from her familiar church and schools and experienced the unanticipated death of a close childhood friend. There was no doubt that a combination of oestrogen dominance, elevated cortisol levels and insufficient DHEA levels were all contributing to why Shirley was packing those pounds around her middle.

I explained to Shirley that oestrogen dominance can cause weight gain and bloating, and that deep abdominal tissue has up to four times the number of cortisol receptors than any other area of the body. When the body is under stress, the cells in the abdomen are the most aggressive in responding to increased cortisol levels. The result is a biochemically driven accumulation of extra abdominal flab.

Six months after her first consultation, Shirley returned and said the following:

> When I first came to you complaining that my gut had become a fat magnet, you recommended that I start a regimen that would include bio-identical progesterone cream, foods and supplements to support hormone balance, and a practice of consciously relaxing three times a day. I bought into your approach to eliminating my condition of oestrogen dominance, but I thought the whole idea of de-stressing to support hormone balance was hokey, so I just blew that part off.

In two months I lost 8 pounds (3.6 kilograms) and was excited. Then for the next two months, no more weight loss. I was discouraged, but I remembered what you had said about how stress can sabotage hormone balance, so I decided to give relaxation a try. I began to practice conscious breathing every time I came to a red light. Also, I set aside ten minutes every morning to just sit quietly and imagine myself at the beach. In four weeks, those last 7 pounds I wanted to lose just melted away.

how stressed are you?

The list shown in Table 6-1 overleaf is adapted from the work of mental health experts Thomas H Holmes and Richard H Rahe. It's very useful for obtaining a snapshot of your overall stress level.

Note that each stress-inducing event has been assigned a life-change unit (LCU). To quantify your stress level, first circle all the life events that you have experienced within the last twelve months. Next, add up the corresponding LCUs. Once you have your LCU total, find your stress-level category. Finally, read how your stress level is linked with hormone imbalance.

Table 6-1. Stress-Inducing Events

Life Event	LCU	Life Event	LCU
Death of spouse	100	Children leaving home	29
Divorce	73	Trouble with difficult teenagers	29
Marital separation	65	Outstanding personal achievement	28
Prison sentence	63	Spouse begins or stops work	26
Death of a close family member	63	Starting or ending school	26
Personal injury or illness	53	Change in living conditions	25
Marriage	50	Revision of personal habits (dress, manners, associations)	24
Being fired from work	47		
Reconciliation with spouse	45	Trouble with boss	23
Retirement	45	Change in work hours or conditions	20
Change in health of a family member	44		
Illness or change in care needs of a parent	40	Change in residence	20
		Change in school	20
Sexual difficulties	39	Change in recreational activities	19
Addition of a family member	39	Change in religious activities	19
Major business readjustment	39	Change in social activities	18
Major change in financial state	38	Mortgage or loan under £10,000	17
Death of a close friend	37	Change in sleeping habits	16
Changing to a different line of work	36	Change in number of family gatherings	15
Change in frequency of arguments with spouse	35		
		Change in eating habits	15
New loan for major purchase over £10,000	31	Holiday	13
		Christmas	12
Foreclosure on a mortgage or loan	30	Minor violation of the law	11
Major change in responsibilities at work	29	LCU Total Score: _____	

Here is what your LCU total score reveals:

- If your total is 0–150: At the moment, your stress level is low. The chance of your stress triggering a hormone imbalance is also low. Good for you.
- If your total is 150–300: You have borderline high stress. Your risk for a stress-related hormone imbalance is moderate.
- If your total is more than 300: Warning! You have a high stress level. Your chance of having a stress-related hormone imbalance is significant.

Because the average person's life is full of responsibilities and complications, it is just not reasonable to think that you can completely eliminate stress as a factor. There are, however, tools and strategies that can help you to better cope with day-to-day stress. Proactive stress management has been shown to decrease the body's susceptibility to the fight-or-flight surge of adrenal hormones.

hormone-healthy habit: beat stress

Although de-stressing is part of the prescription for restoring and maintaining hormone balance, setting aside time for yourself will be one of your greatest challenges. Experiment with different approaches to determine which ones will work best for you.

breathe

A common response to our hurried and fragmented lives is physical tension in the body and shallow breathing through the chest. Simply making a conscious effort to breathe more deeply and slowly can elicit a relaxation response to counteract your automatic stress response.

Try to set aside five minutes three times a day to close your door, take the phone off the hook and just focus on inhalation and exhalation. Some people accomplish this best when they are naturally sequestered; for instance, in a car or on the toilet. Try the following technique:

- Put your hand under your belly button and focus on moving your breath down through your belly rather than up through your chest.
- Breathe in through your nose for a count of four.
- Hold for a count of three.
- Exhale through your mouth for a count of four.

Take any routine interruption that you find annoying in life and 'reprogram' it as a cue to pause and breathe more consciously. Red lights, e-mail message alerts and being put on hold during a telephone call can all serve this function.

meditate

For most of us, our minds are busy even when our bodies are still. When you use meditation to elicit the relaxation response, you turn your attention inward, concentrating on a repetitive positive thought, prayer or image to reduce the reactivity of your thoughts.

Some patients have told me that they meditate by repeating a mantra of love or peace with each exhalation; others say that they recite a memorised prayer; or personally, I picture myself on the shores of a beach listening to the ebb and flow of the waves. I encourage you to develop your own personal meditation to help your body and mind begin to quiet down so that a state of physiological and mental rest can ensue.

Begin by setting aside ten minutes each day to meditate. Do your best to find a quiet space where you won't be disturbed. You can meditate in any position, but the best way is to sit up with a straight back or in a comfortable chair. To help you fully relax and eliminate the need to look at your watch, set a timer or gentle alarm.

visualise

A psychologist I know well has a fun technique to reduce your reaction to stressful people. He suggests that whenever you are around someone who is causing you to tense up or feel anxious, you should visualise that person's face on a tiny mouse's body with really big ears. Then, he suggests, imagine yourself taking a big broom to firmly and efficiently swish that mouse away.

Another visualisation technique is to imagine that your stress has a shape and form and has attached itself like chewing gum to the bottom of your shoe. Visualise yourself taking off your shoe, peeling off that nasty stress and throwing it in the bin. The goal is to create an image of stress as something you can get rid of.

Finally, simply close your eyes and take yourself on a trip to the most peaceful place you have ever been or read about. Imagine how the air feels against your skin and how restful your mind is while you are there. When you reenter your true surroundings, you will most likely feel refreshed from your brief mental holiday.

sleep disturbances and your hormones

Stress can cause you to toss and turn at night. Stress-induced insomnia can impact two hormones that function to stimulate and control your appetite: ghrelin, the hormone that pumps through your body when you feel hungry, and leptin, the hormone that tells you that you are full and to stop eating.

In the long-term Wisconsin Sleep Cohort Study, men and women who routinely slept eight hours nightly were compared to those who slept five hours or less. The findings indicated that those sleeping five hours or less had a 15 per cent higher level of ghrelin, the hormone signalling hunger, and a 16 per cent lower level of leptin, the hormone signalling fullness.

According to Peter Kilpton, health journalist and author of *Less Sleep Can Equal More Weight*, when you are deprived of sleep, the production of ghrelin and leptin are affected, and not in a positive way. Researchers have concluded that a sleep deficit leads to elevated levels of ghrelin in your system. If you are not getting enough sleep, your body responds by telling you that you are hungrier. Furthermore, when you do eat, it will take you longer to feel full and satisfied. This is because the amount of leptin in your system has decreased. The combination of elevated ghrelin (making you feel constantly hungry) and decreased leptin (telling you that you still aren't full) will wreak havoc on your waistline.

hormone-healthy habit: snooze and lose

Substantial medical evidence suggests that there is a strong link between sleep and weight. Researchers say that how much you sleep, and quite possibly the quality of your sleep, can silently orchestrate a symphony of hormonal activity that is tied to your appetite.

According to Michael Breus, a faculty member of the Atlanta School of Sleep Medicine and director of the Sleep Disorders Centers of Southeastern Lung Care in Atlanta, US, a lack of sleep drives leptin levels down, which means that you don't feel as satisfied after you eat. It also causes ghrelin levels to rise, which means that your appetite is stimulated, so you want more food.

Because oestrogen dominance frequently causes insomnia or fitful sleeping as a result of hot flushes and night sweats, using bio-identical progesterone cream and eating foods to reduce your oestrogen load should help to promote a healthy sleeping pattern. However, you still have to make the choice to stop whatever you are doing and get into bed early enough to allow yourself eight hours of sleep.

physical inactivity and your hormones

Numerous studies in the last several decades have confirmed that physical activity has a positive effect on longevity and mortality and that a lack of physical activity is associated with an increased risk of disease and disability. Regular physical activity helps to regulate cortisol production, making it less likely that surging cortisol levels will contribute to both a constant feeling of anxiety and an ever-expanding waistline.

hormone-healthy habit: find a way to move

In order to commit yourself to a regular fitness programme, you must set goals that you know you can meet. If you do not currently exercise, start by planning to simply move your body thirty to forty minutes each day. Do something you enjoy: walk, dance, ride a bike, swim, do yoga, attend an aerobics class or skip. This might sound harsh, but *if you are too busy to exercise every day, then every day you are busy dying*.

boosting your adrenal glands

The adrenal glands are the main site of stress damage in the body. Certain supplements can nourish depleted adrenal glands while encouraging adrenal cortex secretions, which help to maintain optimal hormone balance.

In addition to the supplements described in Chapter 5, I designed an Adrenal Boost formula to increase overall energy and decrease fatigue. It is helpful for people who are under stress because it supports the glands that are responsible for energy flow. Anyone whose adrenal system is depressed by stress should also take 7-keto DHEA.

The ingredients in the Adrenal Boost formula are vitamin C, vitamin B_6, pantothenic acid, deglycerised liquorice root, Mexican wild yam root, schizandra berry, *Eleutherococcus senticosus* root, stinging nettle leaf, trimethylglycine, special plant cellulose, natural silica, vegetable stearate and magnesium stearate. I recommend that people dealing with chronic (long-term) stress take one capsule every morning and every night if they need it.

You should not take Adrenal Boost, however, if you have high blood pressure, because liquorice root can elevate blood pressure.

In summary, you do not have to allow stress and/or poor lifestyle choices to upset your hormone balance. A proactive regime of self-care is the best way to vaporise those weight-loss saboteurs that lurk in the corners of your everyday life. Even though most of us can't take a week a month just to chill out and can't afford a full-time housekeeper, chauffeur or chef, we can make simple (and free) adjustments in our everyday lives to manage daily stress, enjoy a good night's sleep, get some exercise and supplement a fatigued adrenal system.

Hormone balance is a process, not a fixed state. What works to balance your hormones in your thirties and early forties might not work as you approach your late forties and early fifties. The production of your hormones will continue to shift and decline with age.

About 80 per cent of women and men will never need anything more than over-the-counter bio-identical progesterone, our recommended regime of foods and supplements, and a practice of hormone-healthy life habits to maintain optimal hormone balance. However, with age, approximately 20 per cent of women and men will suffer a decline in oestrogen and/or testosterone production that will require treatment. They will need the help of a knowledgeable physician and a compounding pharmacist. For those who are on a comprehensive bio-identical hormone replacement regime, it will be critical that they stick to their diet and take their supplements if they want to lose their belly fat and keep it off for good.

THE 80-20 RULE　⑦

I n this chapter I introduce you to what I call the 80-20 rule of bio-identical hormone replacement therapy (BHRT) and long-term weight management. Approximately 80 per cent of men and women find that over-the-counter bio-identical progesterone cream, combined with foods and supplements to support hormone balance, is all they need to get and keep those unwanted pounds off. However, the other 20 per cent discover that the pounds begin to creep back on and realise that they need a bit more help.

How will you know if you are one of the 20 per cent who needs extra bio-identical hormone support? Your body will tell you. Typically, this will happen in your late forties and fifties.

Pam had been my patient for twelve years. When she first came in at the age of thirty-nine, she was 25 pounds (11 kilograms) overweight and experiencing constant headaches, fatigue and bloating. After following the three-step plan for just a month, her symptoms went away. She lost all the excess weight in four months and, by continuing on the plan, kept those pounds off. Then, when she was fifty-one years old, Pam was back in the office for her annual exam, and she wasn't happy.

'What has happened to your bio-identical progesterone cream?' she asked. 'I am still eating all the foods to reduce my oestrogen load and taking my supplements, but I have gained 19 pounds (5 kilograms) in nine months. It's got to be a change in your cream!'

Pam complained that she was having night sweats and hot flushes. She also reported that she had not had a period for eleven months. When a woman has not had a period for twelve months, she is officially menopausal. Pam was on that cusp, and the production of her other sex hormones had declined to a point that additional help might be necessary. The progesterone cream had not changed, but the balance among her other hormones had.

one size does not fit all

As stated in the previous chapter, hormone balance is a process, not a fixed state. Although progesterone production is the first to decline in women, with age the production of oestrogen and testosterone will also decline. This means that the hormone replacement that works for you today might not work for you five years from now.

How will you know if you are one of the 20 per cent who also needs to address a shift in oestrogen and testosterone production? Your symptoms will be your first clue. If symptoms of hormone imbalance persist or return when you are using a regime of bio-identical progesterone cream and foods and supplements to support hormone balance, then the balance of your other hormones has also shifted and will require attention.

Women in their thirties or forties who enter abrupt artificial menopause as a result of a complete hysterectomy should be placed on a full regime of bio-identical hormone replacement. As they age, some women sail through natural menopause with the help of the three-step plan only. Other women have a flare-up of symptoms that require additional hormone supplementation. As for men, if they experience a progressive decline in libido in their late forties and early fifties, they should work with a doctor to determine if they are candidates for bio-identical testosterone replacement.

when you will need a doctor

A doctor will have to order either a saliva or a blood serum test to analyse all your hormone levels. Once a doctor has determined which hormones are deficient, he or she may be able to write a prescription for a formulation of BHRT to address your unique needs.

Patients come to see me from all over the world because it's not always easy to find a doctor who has experience diagnosing hormone imbalances and BHRT as the preferred treatment. BHRT is not yet taught in medical schools, and most doctors remain uneducated about it.

However, since the World Health Institute has begun detailing the significant health risks of synthetic hormone replacement, this trend is shifting. In the last several years, hundreds of doctors in the US have attended national continuing medical education forums on the subject of BHRT. In most cases, these doctors have been prodded by their patients' demands for safe and effective alternatives; as a result, these doctors have taken the initiative to educate themselves.

If you do not know a doctor in your area who is proficient in BHRT, see www.npis.info for more information.

Once your doctor determines exactly which hormones are deficient, your prescription will have to be filled in a compounding pharmacy. Although some pharmaceutical companies are now manufacturing standard dosages of BHRT, it is more typical for a doctor to write a prescription for the exact amount of the hormones that your body needs. A compounding pharmacist will then mix your individualised prescription on site.

If you have never had your prescriptions filled by a compounding pharmacist, here are some facts you should know:

- Every compounding pharmacy is licensed and inspected by the State Pharmacy Board.
- Compounding pharmacists are educated and trained to provide information about the formulation of bio-identical hormones. In many cases, they help to educate the physician on dosing and delivery options.
- All materials used in compounding formulations are

subject to FDA (in the US) inspection and the agency's Good Manufacturing Procedures code.

- The International Academy of Compounding Pharmacists (IACP) and the Professional Compounding Centers for America (PCCA) are two excellent resources to help you or your physician locate a compounding pharmacy in your area. Their contact information is provided in Appendix C.

If you are one of the 20 per cent who require a more comprehensive plan of BHRT, you will still need help to win your battle of the bulge. Also remember: you should never take any form of oestrogen therapy, even if it is bio-identical, without also taking bio-identical progesterone.

If you are on any form of bio-identical oestrogen replacement, it might seem counterproductive to continue to eat foods and take supplements to reduce your oestrogen load. However, it is not. In fact, by continuing to eat foods that reduce your oestrogen load and take supplements that support overall hormone balance, you can positively influence how the oestrogen is metabolised in your body.

The names for the three most commonly prescribed formulations of bio-identical oestrogen are tri-est, bi-est and oestradiol. Tri-est is a combination of the three oestrogens you learned about earlier: oestrone (E1), oestradiol (E2) and oestriol (E3). Bi-est is a combination of E2 and E3, and oestradiol is simple E2. Just like the oestrogen produced by your ovaries, bio-identical oestrogen returns to the liver to be metabolised after it completes its required activity within the body. There it is broken down into different enzymatic pathways. The first, the 2-hydroxy pathway, results in 'good' oestrogen metabolites. The second, the 16-hydroxy pathway, produces one of the 'bad' oestrogen metabolites, which results in an increased risk of cancer. The third, the 4-hydroxy pathway, is associated with an even higher rate of cancer.

It seems obvious that you should want more 'good' oestrogens than 'bad' oestrogens. Foods and supplements can influence which enzymatic pathway oestrogen goes down. For instance, you have learned that cruciferous vegetables act as a catalyst to pull oestrogen down a benign pathway to 2-hydroxyestrone, thus decreasing the levels of the carcinogenic 4- and 16-alpha hydroxyestrones, the 'bad' oestrogens. In addition, the supplement DIM supports the activity of enzymes that improve oestrogen metabolism by increasing the levels of 2-hydroxyestrone, the 'good' oestrogen.

If you are on a more comprehensive BHRT regime that includes bio-identical oestrogen, it is essential that you stick to this plan. When you do, you will continue to reduce your unhealthy oestrogen load, support overall hormone balance, protect yourself from hormone-dependent cancers and keep your belly flat for life.

THE 'FLAT BELLY FOR LIFE' RECIPE COLLECTION

MAIN DISHES

Asparagus Omelette

4 egg whites
¼ teaspoon salt
4 egg yolks
Dash of pepper
225 ml (4 fl oz) low-fat cottage cheese
1½ tablespoons extra-virgin olive oil
6 asparagus spears, trimmed and slightly
    steamed

Preheat oven to 180°C/350°F/gas mark 4. Beat egg whites until frothy. Add salt and beat until stiff. Beat yolks until thick and lemon coloured; add pepper and cottage cheese and beat until well blended. Fold egg whites into yolks. Heat olive oil in a 25-centimetre (10-inch) iron frying pan; pour in omelette and cook approximately 3 minutes, until the bottom is lightly browned. Top with asparagus spears and finish cooking in the oven for 15 minutes or until a knife inserted in the centre comes out clean. Makes 2 servings.

NUTRITION FACTS

Amount Per Serving: Calories 340 – Calories from Fat 190 – Total Fat 21 g
Saturated Fat 6 g – Cholesterol 420 mg – Sodium 840 mg – Total Carbohydrate 11 g
Dietary Fibre 2 g – Sugars 7 g – Protein 26 g – Calcium 25% DV

Baked Fish with Basil

Organic non-stick cooking spray
6 x 175 g (6 oz) fish fillets
40 g (1½ oz) fresh basil, chopped
60 ml (2 fl oz) extra-virgin olive oil
2 tablespoons minced garlic
1 tablespoon lemon juice
Salt and pepper to taste
1 lemon, sliced

Preheat oven to 180°C/350°F/gas mark 4. Place fish fillets in baking dish that you've sprayed with organic non-stick cooking spray. Combine basil, olive oil, garlic and lemon juice in small bowl. Mix well and spoon evenly over fish. Add salt and pepper. Bake for 20–25 minutes, until the fish flakes easily with a fork. Garnish with lemon slices and serve. Makes 6 servings.

NUTRITION FACTS

Amount Per Serving: Calories 250 – Calories from Fat 110 – Total Fat 12 g
Saturated Fat 2.5 g – Cholesterol 85 mg – Sodium 90 mg – Total Carbohydrate 1 g
Dietary Fibre 0 g – Sugars 0 g – Protein 35 g – Calcium 4% DV

Black Beanofritos

450 g (16 oz) canned black beans
1 medium tomato, chopped
1 small onion, minced
Salt and pepper to taste
1 avocado
100 g (3½ oz) natural low-fat yoghurt
4 low-fat wholemeal tortilla wraps
2 tablespoons chopped fresh coriander
Dash of Tabasco hot sauce (optional)

In a medium frying pan, sauté the black beans with the tomato and onion until the vegetables are soft and the beans are hot. Add salt and pepper while mixture is cooking. Peel the avocado, mash with a potato masher and mix well with yoghurt. Remove bean mixture from frying pan and drain any liquid. Using the potato masher, mash the bean mixture and then spoon it evenly onto the centre of each tortilla, placed on a plate or platter. Fold the tortilla over, top with with a tablespoon of the avocado-yoghurt mixture and sprinkle with fresh coriander (and a dash of Tabasco hot sauce if desired) before serving. Makes 4 servings.

NUTRITION FACTS

Amount Per Serving: Calories 340 – Calories from Fat 90 – Total Fat 9 g – Saturated Fat 1 g – Cholesterol 0 mg – Sodium 190 mg – Total Carbohydrate 51 g Dietary Fibre 11 g – Sugars 4 g – Protein 14 g – Calcium 6% DV

Cauliflower and Turkey Bacon Soup

425 g (15 oz) white onion, chopped

3 tablespoons extra-virgin olive oil

2 teaspoons ground cumin

1½ teaspoons ground fennel

400 g (14 oz) brown rice

1 litre (1¾ pints) hot water

575 g (1 lb 4½ oz) cauliflower, chopped

115 g (4 oz) carrots, grated

1 bouillon cube

2 tablespoons fresh lemon juice

Salt and pepper to taste

5 rashers cooked turkey bacon, crumbled

In a large soup pan on medium heat, sauté the onion in the olive oil for 5–10 minutes until translucent. Stir in the cumin, fennel and brown rice. Add hot water. Cover and bring to the boil. Add the cauliflower, carrots and bouillon and return to the boil before lowering the heat to simmer for 10–15 minutes. Remove from heat.

In a blender, purée the vegetables and broth until smooth. Add the lemon juice and salt and pepper. Return to soup pan and reheat. Top with crumbled turkey bacon just before serving. Makes 6–8 servings.

NUTRITION FACTS

Amount Per Serving: Calories 310 – Calories from Fat 100 – Total Fat 11 g
Saturated Fat 2 g – Cholesterol 10 mg – Sodium 420 mg – Total Carbohydrate 44 g
Dietary Fibre 7 g – Sugars 7 g – Protein 9 g – Calcium 6% DV

Cauliflower Crab Cakes

275 g (9¾ oz) crabmeat
225 g (8 oz) cooked cauliflower, mashed
40 g (1½ oz) celery, minced
80 g (2¾ oz) onion, minced
1 tablespoon parsley
2 eggs, beaten
Extra-virgin olive oil or grapeseed oil (for
    sautéing)

Combine all ingredients in a large bowl, except the olive oil. Form into 6 patties and chill in refrigerator for at least 1 hour. Brown in frying pan lightly coated with olive oil. Makes 6 servings.

NUTRITION FACTS

Amount Per Serving: Calories 160 – Calories from Fat 40 – Total Fat 4.5 g – Saturated Fat 1 g – Cholesterol 140 mg – Sodium 500 mg – Total Carbohydrate 6 g Dietary Fibre 2 g – Sugars 2 g – Protein 24 g – Calcium 10% DV

Chicken and Asparagus Lettuce Wraps

140 g (5 oz) asparagus, washed and trimmed
4 x 175 g (6 oz) skinless, boneless chicken
   breast halves
2 tablespoons extra-virgin olive oil
1 tablespoon rice vinegar
1 tablespoon low-sodium soya sauce
1 teaspoon grated fresh ginger
½ teaspoon grated orange rind
2 teaspoons minced garlic
½ cup grated carrots
1 head cos lettuce

Chop the asparagus into pieces that are, at most, 75-millimetre (⅓ inch) long. Slice the chicken breast into thin strips. Mix the olive oil, vinegar, soya sauce, ginger, orange rind and garlic in a bowl. Add the chicken and asparagus and chill for 1 hour. Pour into a frying pan, add carrots and brown for 10–12 minutes, until the chicken is done. Drop a large spoonful of the cooked mixture on to the centre of each lettuce leaf. Roll like a burrito and serve. Makes 6 servings.

NUTRITION FACTS

Amount Per Serving: Calories 250 – Calories from Fat 80 – Total Fat 9 g – Saturated Fat 2 g – Cholesterol 95 mg – Sodium 190 mg – Total Carbohydrate 4 g Dietary Fibre 1 g – Sugars 2 g – Protein 36 g – Calcium 4% DV

Colourful Turkey Casserole

1.3 kg (3 lb) turkey breast
1 teaspoon salt
½ teaspoon pepper
½ teaspoon oregano
½ teaspoon rosemary
Extra-virgin olive oil
225 g (8 oz) carrots, grated
275 g (9¾ oz) asparagus, chopped
1 yellow pepper, sliced
450 g (16 oz) passata
2 cloves garlic
360 g (12½ oz) spinach, steamed

Preheat oven to 160°C/325°F/gas mark 3. Cut turkey into strips. Sprinkle with salt, pepper, oregano and rosemary, then brown in a frying pan in olive oil. Place the pieces in a baking dish that is very lightly greased with olive oil. Sauté carrots, asparagus and yellow pepper in frying pan until soft. Remove from heat and stir in passata, garlic and spinach. Pour over chicken and toss. Bake uncovered for 1 hour. Makes 6 servings.

NUTRITION FACTS

Amount Per Serving: Calories 440 – Calories from Fat 20 – Total Fat 2.5 g
Saturated Fat 0.5 g – Cholesterol 190 mg – Sodium 980 mg – Total Carbohydrate 28 g
Dietary Fibre 6 g – Sugars 7 g – Protein 75 g – Calcium 25% DV

Favourite Feta Frittata

450 g (1 lb) spinach leaves, washed and
  chopped
9 large eggs
2 tablespoons skimmed milk
40 g (1½ oz) Parmesan cheese, grated
2 tablespoons chopped sun-dried tomatoes
Salt and freshly ground pepper to taste
1 medium onion, chopped
1 tablespoon extra-virgin olive oil
1 large clove garlic, minced
85 g (3 oz) reduced-fat feta cheese

Preheat oven to 200°C/400°F/gas mark 6. Cook
spinach in 60 ml (2 oz) water in covered saucepan until just
wilted (a couple of minutes). Drain water and set aside. In
a mixing bowl, whisk together eggs, milk and Parmesan
cheese. Add tomatoes and sprinkle with salt and pepper.
Set aside.

Sauté onion in olive oil in an oven-safe frying pan until translucent, about 2 minutes on medium-high heat. Add garlic and
sauté a minute more. Add cooked spinach and mix with onion
and garlic. Spread spinach mixture evenly on the base of the frying pan. Pour the egg mixture over the spinach mixture. Use a
spatula to lift up the spinach mixture along the sides of the pan
to let the egg mixture flow underneath. Sprinkle bits of feta
cheese over the top of the frittata mixture.

When the mixture is about half set, put the whole pan in the oven. Bake 13–15 minutes, until frittata is puffy and golden. Remove from oven and allow to cool for several minutes. Makes 5 servings.

NUTRITION FACTS

Amount Per Serving: Calories 250 – Calories from Fat 150 – Total Fat 16 g
Saturated Fat 6 g – Cholesterol 390 mg – Sodium 540 mg – Total Carbohydrate 7 g
Dietary Fibre 3 g – Sugars 3 g – Protein 20 g – Calcium 25% DV

Fish New Orleans Style

3 bay leaves
3 sprigs fresh thyme or 1 tablespoon dried thyme
1 clove garlic
½ teaspoon salt
½ teaspoon pepper
A pinch of cayenne pepper
1.3 kg (3 lb) whitefish, such as plaice
   or hake
70 g (2½ oz) broccoli, chopped
175 g (6 oz) tomatoes, chopped
50 g (1¾ oz) spring onions, chopped
Extra-virgin olive oil
1 lemon

Preheat oven to 180°C/350°F/gas mark 4. Chop bay leaves, thyme and garlic very fine. Add salt, pepper and cayenne. Rub the fish inside and out with this mixture and place in a baking dish. Sauté the broccoli, tomatoes and spring onions in olive oil. Pour over fish and bake for 30 minutes. Squeeze lemon on to fish before serving. Makes 6 servings.

NUTRITION FACTS

Amount Per Serving: Calories 220 – Calories from Fat 25 – Total Fat 3 g – Saturated Fat 0.5 g – Cholesterol 110 mg – Sodium 390 mg – Total Carbohydrate 4 g Dietary Fibre 1 g – Sugars 1 g – Protein 43 g – Calcium 6% DV

Garlic Chickpeas and Pasta

450 g (16 oz) canned chickpeas
225 g (8 oz) canned chopped tomatoes with
    basil
115 g (4 oz) steamed broccoli, chopped
3 tablespoons chopped garlic
225 ml (8 fl oz) water
½ teaspoon extra-virgin olive oil
Salt and pepper to taste
225 g (8 oz) uncooked wholemeal pasta

In large bowl, mix chickpeas, tomatoes, broccoli and garlic. Add water, olive oil, salt and pepper to a large pot and bring to the boil. Add pasta and cook according to the time recommended on the packet. Remove pasta, drain and toss with chickpea mixture. Serve immediately. Makes 6 servings.

NUTRITION FACTS

Amount Per Serving: Calories 210 – Calories from Fat 25 – Total Fat 2.5 g – Saturated Fat 0 g – Cholesterol 0 mg – Sodium 135 mg – Total Carbohydrate 39 g Dietary Fibre 9 g – Sugars 6 g – Protein 11 g – Calcium 6% DV

Fish with Citrus Marinade

60 ml (2 fl oz) extra-virgin olive oil
2 tablespoons grapefruit juice
3 tablespoons lime juice
Salt and pepper to taste
4 x 175 g (6 oz) fish fillets

Combine olive oil, grapefruit juice, lime juice, salt and pepper. Pour over fish and marinate in refrigerateor for 2 or more hours. Grill or barbecue and serve. Makes 4 servings.

NUTRITION FACTS

Amount Per Serving: Calories 200 – Calories from Fat 60 – Total Fat 6 g – Saturated Fat 1.5 g – Cholesterol 85 mg – Sodium 90 mg – Total Carbohydrate 0 g Dietary Fibre 0 g – Sugars 0 g – Protein 34 g – Calcium 2% DV

Salmon with Dill and Lemon

2 tablespoons dill
1 teaspoon garlic powder
4 tablespoons extra-virgin olive oil
2 tablespoons white wine vinegar
   with tarragon
Juice of 2 lemons
4 x 2.5-cm-thick (1-inch) each salmon steaks,
   115 g (4 oz)

Mix dill, garlic powder, olive oil, vinegar and lemon juice. Pour mixture over salmon steaks and marinate in the refrigerator for at least 2 hours, turning at least once. Place salmon on hot barbecue or griddle pan and cook 3–5 minutes on each side. Makes 4 servings.

NUTRITION FACTS

Amount Per Serving: Calories 280 – Calories from Fat 130 – Total Fat 14 g
Saturated Fat 2 g – Cholesterol 95 mg – Sodium 75 mg – Total Carbohydrate 1 g
Dietary Fibre 0 g – Sugars 0 g – Protein 34 g – Calcium 2% DV

Lemon Hot Fish

Organic non-stick cooking spray
6 x 115 g (4 oz) fillets of whitefish
5 cloves garlic, chopped
50 g (1¾ oz) fresh spinach
85 g (3 oz) cauliflower, sliced thin
2–3 bay leaves
225 ml (8 fl oz) lemon juice
125 ml (4 fl oz) rice wine vinegar
2 tablespoons Tabasco hot sauce
2 tablespoons extra-virgin olive oil
Salt and pepper to taste
2 tablespoons toasted flaxseed
1 lemon cut into wedges
Fresh parsley

Preheat oven to 180°C/350°F/gas mark 4. Place fish in
a baking tin that you've sprayed with organic non-stick
cooking spray. Cover with garlic, spinach, cauliflower and
bay leaves. In a small bowl, mix the lemon juice, vinegar,
Tabasco hot sauce, olive oil, salt and pepper. Pour over
fish. Bake covered for 30 minutes, stirring vegetables twice
so they absorb the juice evenly. Then bake uncovered for
another 15 minutes. Remove and place on serving platter.
Remove bay leaves. Sprinkle with toasted flaxseed and garnish with lemons and parsley. Makes 6 servings.

NUTRITION FACTS

Amount Per Serving: Calories 160 – Calories from Fat 45 – Total Fat 5 g – Saturated
Fat 1 g – Cholesterol 55 mg – Sodium 75 mg – Total Carbohydrate 4 g
Dietary Fibre 2 g – Sugars 1 g – Protein 24 g – Calcium 4% DV

Lentil, Carrot and Turnip Stew

190 g (6¾ oz) red lentils
4 large carrots, sliced
1–2 large onions, chopped
1 tablespoon minced garlic
Extra-virgin olive oil
450 g (16 oz) canned tomatoes or 8–10 fresh
   ones, chopped
450 g (16 oz) frozen chopped turnips
2–3 sprigs parsley or 1 teaspoon dried parsley
Salt, pepper and Tabasco hot sauce to taste

Thoroughly rinse the red lentils in a sieve and remove any small black rocks that are sometimes found among them. Boil the lentils in a large pot for about 20 minutes, in enough water so that the lentils can expand to roughly four times their original size. Add carrots and boil for 5 more minutes. Brown the onion and garlic in olive oil in a frying pan. Add onion mixture to the pot. Toss in the can of tomatoes (with the liquid) and add the turnips and parsley. Cook over low to medium heat for 15 minutes, stirring occasionally so the lentils don't stick to the base of the pan. Add salt, pepper and Tabasco hot sauce to taste. Serve in bowls. Makes 4 servings.

NUTRITION FACTS

Amount Per Serving: Calories 260 – Calories from Fat 15 – Total Fat 1.5 g – Saturated Fat 0 g – Cholesterol 0 mg – Sodium 115 mg – Total Carbohydrate 52 g Dietary Fibre 17 g – Sugars 20 g – Protein 15 g – Calcium 15% DV

Nest of Beans and Greens

155 g (5½ oz) dried butter beans
2 hard-boiled eggs, finely chopped
3 tablespoons extra-virgin olive oil
1 bunch of turnip, spring or mustard greens
    (about 900 g/2 lbs) or 450 g (16 oz) frozen
    greens
Juice of 1 lemon
Salt, pepper, vinegar and crushed pepper flakes
    (optional) to taste

Soak and cook butter beans according to the directions on the packet. Drain. Add the eggs to the beans and use a potato masher to mash into a paste. Use the olive oil sparingly if some moisture is needed. Set aside. Sauté the greens in a medium saucepan until tender but still green. Make a nest of greens on each plate. Put 2 tablespoons of the butter bean mash in the centre. Sprinkle lemon juice and season as desired with salt, pepper, vinegar and red pepper flakes. Makes 4 servings.

NUTRITION FACTS

Amount Per Serving: Calories 310 – Calories from Fat 130 – Total Fat 14 g
Saturated Fat 2.5 g – Cholesterol 105 mg – Sodium 85 mg – Total Carbohydrate 35 g
Dietary Fibre 15 g – Sugars 1 g – Protein 16 g – Calcium 35% DV

Open-Faced Veggie Cheeseburger

115 g (4 oz) green beans
85 g (3 oz) cracked wheat
1 small courgette
1 small carrot, peeled
½ Granny Smith apple, peeled
240 g (8½ oz) canned chickpeas, rinsed and
    drained
1 tablespoon minced onion
1 tablespoon minced garlic
½ teaspoon curry powder
½ teaspoon chilli powder
Salt and pepper to taste
2 tablespoons extra-virgin olive oil
55 g (2 oz) Cheddar cheese, grated
70 g (2½ oz) dried wholemeal breadcrumbs
Sliced tomato, onion and wholemeal
    hamburger buns (optional)

Cook green beans in boiling water until tender but crisp.
Drain and chop very fine. Cook cracked wheat in 225 ml
(8 fl oz) boiling water for 1 minute. Remove from heat and
cover. Grate the courgette, carrot and apple; place on
some kitchen paper and squeeze out excess moisture.
Combine with the chopped beans.

In a food processor, blend the chickpeas, onions, garlic,
curry powder, chilli powder, salt, pepper and olive oil until
smooth. Add to the green bean mixture.

Drain the cracked wheat in a sieve, pressing with the back of a spoon to extract excess liquid. Add to the vegetables. Stir in the cheese and add the breadcrumbs. Refrigerate for 1 hour.

Shape into four burgers. Cook 3 minutes on each side on a hot barbecue or grill lightly brushed with olive oil. Serve as is or on ½ hamburger bun; top with tomato and onion if desired. Makes 4 servings.

NUTRITION FACTS

Amount Per Serving: Calories 290 – Calories from Fat 120 – Total Fat 13 g
Saturated Fat 4.5 g – Cholesterol 15 mg – Sodium 200 mg – Total Carbohydrate 33 g
Dietary Fibre 6 g – Sugars 5 g – Protein 10 g – Calcium 15% DV

Orange-Ginger Salmon

225 ml (8 fl oz) extra-virgin olive oil
125 ml (4 fl oz) orange juice
1 tablespoon minced garlic
4 x 150 g (5 oz) salmon steaks, 2.5 cm (1 inch)
   thick
Fresh ginger slivers

Mix the olive oil, orange juice and garlic. Pour the mixture over the salmon and marinate at least 2 hours (or refrigerate overnight). Preheat the grill. Grill the fish 4–7.5 centimetres (2–3 inches) from the heating element for 5 minutes, then turn and grill on the other side. You may also heat any saved marinade and spoon over the fish just before serving. Makes 4 servings.

NUTRITION FACTS

Amount Per Serving: Calories 310 – Calories from Fat 160 – Total Fat 18 g
Saturated Fat 2.5 g – Cholesterol 95 mg – Sodium 75 mg – Total Carbohydrate 2 g
Dietary Fibre 0 g – Sugars 1 g – Protein 34 g – Calcium 2% DV

Pan-Roasted Fish
with Parsley and Turkey Bacon

8 rashers turkey bacon
3 tablespoons extra-virgin olive oil
70 g (2½ oz) baby field mushrooms, sliced
1 tablespoon minced garlic
2 tablespoons minced parsley
4 x 175 g (6 oz) fish fillets (or 680–900 g/
    1½–2 lb whole fish)
Salt and pepper to taste
Lemon wedges

Cut the turkey bacon into 2.5-centimetre (1-inch) pieces and sauté in frying pan in 1 tablespoon olive oil for 2–3 minutes; add the mushrooms and cook about 5 more minutes. Stir in the garlic and parsley and remove from heat. Put the remaining 2 tablespoons of olive oil in a frying pan and add the fish fillets. Cook on low to medium heat for 10–15 minutes or until a fork or knife easily penetrates the flesh. Pour the bacon mixture over the fish and let simmer. Add salt and pepper. Serve immediately and garnish with lemon wedges. Makes 4 servings.

NUTRITION FACTS

Amount Per Serving: Calories 380 – Calories from Fat 190 – Total Fat 21 g
Saturated Fat 5 g – Cholesterol 115 mg – Sodium 740 mg – Total Carbohydrate 3 g
Dietary Fibre 1 g – Sugars 1 g – Protein 43 g – Calcium 2% DV

Quick Turkey-Stuffed Cabbage

450 g (16 oz) turkey mince
1 large onion, chopped
100 g (3¾ oz) brown rice, uncooked
4 tablespoons fresh choppd mint or
   1 tablespoon dried mint
1 egg, beaten
800 g (28 oz) canned chicken broth
Salt and pepper to taste
2 tablespoons extra-virgin olive oil
1 medium cabbage
2 tablespoons flaxseed

Preheat oven to 180°C/350°F/gas mark 4. Combine the turkey, onion, rice, mint, egg, broth, salt and pepper and sauté in olive oil until browned. In another pot, steam the cabbage until it is slightly soft. After the cabbage cools, cut off the base, peel off the leaves and place them in a baking dish one by one. Spoon a helping of turkey mixture on to each leaf and then roll it up. Sprinkle with flaxseed and bake for 15–20 minutes. Makes 8 servings.

NUTRITION FACTS

Amount Per Serving: Calories 290 – Calories from Fat 100 – Total Fat 12 g
Saturated Fat 2.5 g – Cholesterol 70 mg – Sodium 130 mg – Total Carbohydrate 31 g
Dietary Fibre 6 g – Sugars 6 g – Protein 18 g – Calcium 10% DV

Rosemary-Baked Chicken Breast

4 skinless, boneless chicken breasts
2 tablespoons minced garlic
3 tablespoons fresh rosemary or 4 tablespoons
   dried rosemary
2 tablespoon lemon juice
Salt and pepper to taste

Preheat the oven to 190°C/375°F/gas mark 5. Put the chicken breasts in a baking dish and cover them with garlic, then sprinkle with rosemary, lemon juice, salt and pepper. Bake uncovered for 25 minutes. Makes 4 servings.

NUTRITION FACTS

Amount Per Serving: Calories 140 – Calories from Fat 15 – Total Fat 1.5 g – Saturated Fat 0 g – Cholesterol 70 mg – Sodium 80 mg – Total Carbohydrate 2 g Dietary Fibre 0 g – Sugars 0 g – Protein 28 g – Calcium 2% DV

Savoury Spinach and Salmon Salad

3 tablespoons orange juice
2 tablespoons low-sodium soya sauce
2 teaspoons minced fresh ginger
1 teaspoon raw honey
1½ teaspoons extra-virgin olive oil
4 x 175 g (6 oz) salmon fillets
90 g (3¼ oz) fresh spinach, washed
90 g (3¼ oz) mandarin orange slices
35 g (1¼ oz) spring onions, chopped
2 hard-boiled eggs, sliced
25 g (1 oz) ground almonds mixed with
    1 tablespoon ground or milled flaxseed

In a small bowl, combine the orange juice, soya sauce, ginger and honey. Whisk, gradually adding the olive oil, until well blended.

Grill, bake or poach the salmon fillets. Make a bed of spinach on each of four plates. Place salmon in the centre of each one. Garnish each with mandarin orange slices, spring onions and eggs. Drizzle the orange–soya sauce dressing over the entire plate and sprinkle with almond-flaxseed mixture. Makes 4 servings.

NUTRITION FACTS

Amount Per Serving: Calories 370 – Calories from Fat 170 – Total Fat 19 g
Saturated Fat 3 g – Cholesterol 200 mg – Sodium 430 mg – Total Carbohydrate 10 g
Dietary Fibre 2 g – Sugars 6 g – Protein 40 g – Calcium 8% DV

Spicy Kale and Beans

375 g (13 oz) dried black-eyed beans
1 bunch kale (about 900 g/2 lb)
1 large onion, diced
1 tablespoon extra-virgin olive oil
2 tablespoons white vinegar
¼ teaspoon crushed red pepper (optional)
2 hard-boiled eggs, chopped

Soak black-eyed beans overnight. The next day place the drained beans in a large saucepan, cover with water and bring to the boil over high heat. Boil for 3 minutes. Remove the pan from the heat, cover tightly and let stand for 1 hour. Wash kale, remove large stem ends and coarsely chop the leaves.

Sauté the onion in a large frying pan. Add the kale and cook for about 5 minutes, until the leaves are wilted but still bright green. Stir in black-eyed beans, vinegar and crushed red pepper until entire mixture bubbles with heat. Top with the eggs before serving. Makes 8 servings.

NUTRITION FACTS

Amount Per Serving: Calories 200 – Calories from Fat 35 – Total Fat 4 g – Saturated Fat 0.5 g – Cholesterol 55 mg – Sodium 480 mg – Total Carbohydrate 32 g Dietary Fibre 7 g – Sugars 1 g – Protein 11 g – Calcium 20% DV

Tossed Turkey Bacon and Spinach Salad

55 g (2 oz) flaked almonds
1 tablespoon sesame seeds
1 tablespoon flaxseed
8 rashers cooked turkey bacon, chopped
90 g (¾ oz) raw spinach, washed
4 spring onions, chopped fine

Dressing
4 tablespoons extra-virgin olive oil
2 tablespoons Worcestershire sauce
2 teaspoons garlic paste or crushed garlic
4 tablespoons lemon juice
1 raw egg
¾ teaspoon salt
¾ teaspoon pepper

Preheat oven to 180°C/350°F/gas mark 4. Roast almonds, sesame seeds and flaxseed for 3–5 minutes. Set aside. Mix turkey bacon, spinach and spring onions in a small bowl. Put the dressing ingredients in a blender and blend until well mixed. Toss the salad with the dressing. Sprinkle with nut-seed mix just before serving. Makes 2 servings.

NUTRITION FACTS

Amount Per Serving: Calories 740 – Calories from Fat 560 – Total Fat 62 g
Saturated Fat 11 g – Cholesterol 160 mg – Sodium 2420 mg – Total Carbohydrate 19 g
Dietary Fibre 6 g – Sugars 5 g – Protein 28 g – Calcium 20% DV

Tuna Melt

350 g (12 oz) canned albacore tuna in water
2 tablespoons natural low-fat yoghurt
1 hard-boiled egg, chopped
1 tablespoon minced fresh parsley
Salt and pepper to taste
4 slices wholemeal bread
1 tomato, sliced
55 g (2 oz) skimmed milk mozzarella, grated

Drain tuna and mix with yoghurt, egg and parsley. Add salt and pepper. Toast the bread in the toaster or under a pre-heated grill; it should be crisp to the touch. Cover the bread generously with tuna mixture, then top with a tomato slice and grated cheese. Pace under a preheated grill and heat until the cheese melts. Makes 4 servings.

NUTRITION FACTS

Amount Per Serving: Calories 190 – Calories from Fat 60 – Total Fat 7 g – Saturated Fat 3 g – Cholesterol 80 mg – Sodium 410 mg – Total Carbohydrate 15 g Dietary Fibre 2 g – Sugars 4 g – Protein 19 g – Calcium 15% DV

Turkey and Asparagus Wraps

16 asparagus spears
100 g (3½ oz) natural low-fat yoghurt
1 teaspoon lemon juice
1 teaspoon curry powder
Salt and pepper to taste
450 g (16 oz) turkey breast slices

Wash, trim and steam asparagus spears until tender. Set aside to cool. Mix yoghurt, lemon juice, curry powder, salt and pepper in a small bowl. Place 2 or 3 slices of turkey breast on a plate. Spread with the yoghurt mixture. Put asparagus spears on one end and roll up. Secure with cocktail stick if necessary. Serve immediately or refrigerate. Makes 4 servings.

NUTRITION FACTS

Amount Per Serving: Calories 140 – Calories from Fat 15 – Total Fat 1.5 g – Saturated Fat 0 g – Cholesterol 50 mg – Sodium 1200 mg – Total Carbohydrate 10 g Dietary Fibre 2 g – Sugars 3 g – Protein 25 g – Calcium 6% DV

Turkey, Apple and Spinach Pitta

2 tablespoons extra-virgin olive oil

2 tablespoons lemon juice

225 g (8 oz) cooked turkey, cut into chunks

1 teaspoon nutmeg, or to taste

Salt and pepper to taste

1 medium apple, cored and thinly sliced

2 pitta bread, separated

Fresh spinach, washed

150 g (5½ oz) natural low-fat yoghurt

Heat olive oil in a frying pan over medium heat. Stir in lemon juice. Mix in turkey; season with nutmeg and salt and pepper. Continue cooking until heated through.

Remove from heat. Stir in apple. Stuff the pittas with fresh spinach leaves and the turkey mixture. Drizzle with yoghurt. Makes 4 servings.

NUTRITION FACTS

Amount Per Serving: Calories 420 – Calories from Fat 80 – Total Fat 9 g – Saturated Fat 2 g – Cholesterol 95 mg – Sodium 410 mg – Total Carbohydrate 40 g Dietary Fibre 2 g – Sugars 5 g – Protein 42 g – Calcium 15% DV

Veggie Burgers

1 medium onion, chopped very fine
1 medium pepper, chopped very fine
Extra-virgin olive oil
90 g (3¼ oz) cooked fresh spinach, drained and
    chopped fine
125 g (4½ oz) Mashed Cauliflower (see recipe
    on page 165)
400 g (14 oz) canned black beans, drained
1 tablespoon garlic powder
1 egg, beaten well
2 pieces wholemeal toast, crumbled fine
Salt and pepper to taste

Sauté onion and pepper in olive oil until onion is translucent. When mixture has cooled, place it in a large bowl
and add all other ingredients, mixing well. Form patties and
place on baking sheet. Chill for at least 2 hours before
browning in olive oil in a frying pan on top of the stove or
bake at 200°C/400°F/gas mark 6 for 30 minutes.
Makes 4 servings.

NUTRITION FACTS

Amount Per Serving: Calories 170 – Calories from Fat 30 – Total Fat 3 g – Saturated
Fat 1 g – Cholesterol 55 mg – Sodium 190 mg – Total Carbohydrate 26 g
Dietary Fibre 7 g – Sugars 5 g – Protein 10 g – Calcium 8% DV

VEGETABLE DISHES

Asian Cabbage

225 g (8 oz) cabbage, finely shredded
115 g (4 oz) carrots, grated
45 g (1½ oz) fresh spinach
2 tablespoons extra-virgin olive oil
1 teaspoon grated fresh ginger
Dash of Tabasco hot sauce (optional)
Lemon juice
1 tablespoon toasted sesame seeds

Stir-fry the cabbage, carrots and spinach in olive oil in a frying pan or wok. Once the vegetables are tender, stir in the grated ginger and Tabasco hot sauce. Before serving, sprinkle with lemon juice. Put on a plate and top with toasted sesame seeds. Makes 6 servings.

NUTRITION FACTS

Amount Per Serving: Calories 60 – Calories from Fat 45 – Total Fat 5 g – Saturated Fat 0.5 g – Cholesterol 0 mg – Sodium 20 mg – Total Carbohydrate 4 g – Dietary Fibre 1 g Sugars 2 g – Protein 1 g – Calcium 4% DV

Baked Swede

Note: Swede is a root vegetable that looks very much like a turnip with yellow-orange flesh and ridges at its neck. This beta carotene-rich vegetable has a delicate sweetness and flavour that hints of the light freshness of cabbage and turnip. With its easy preparation and versatility, great nutrition and excellent flavour, the swede can easily become an endearing family favourite.

2 or 3 medium-sized swedes
4 apples
1 teaspoon olive oil
1 teaspoon salt
⅛ teaspoon white pepper
2 tablespoons butter substitute

Preheat oven to 180°C/350°F/gas mark 4. Peel swedes and apples and slice them 50 millimetre (¼ inch) thick. Use the olive oil to grease the baking dish then sprinkle with salt and pepper and dot with butter. Bake for 25–30 minutes. Makes 8 servings.

NUTRITION FACTS

Amount Per Serving: Calories 110 – Calories from Fat 35 – Total Fat 3.5 g – Saturated Fat 2 g – Cholesterol 10 mg – Sodium 320 mg – Total Carbohydrate 19 g Dietary Fibre 5 g – Sugars 14 g – Protein 2 g – Calcium 8% DV

Beetroot and Brussels Sprouts

4 medium beetroot
10–12 Brussels sprouts
Extra-virgin olive oil
1 small white onion, peeled and sliced thin
3 tablespoons orange juice concentrate
2 teaspoons grated ginger
Salt and pepper to taste

Boil beetroot for 45 minutes or until tender by touch with a fork; drain when done. Remove and discard the outer leaves of the Brussels sprouts and boil them in a separate pan for 5 minutes. Drain and cut in half. Put olive oil in frying pan, sauté onion and add beetroot and Brussels sprouts. Cook until warm, about 2–3 minutes, then stir in orange juice concentrate and ginger. Salt and pepper to taste. Makes 6 servings.

NUTRITION FACTS

Amount Per Serving: Calories 70 – Calories from Fat 15 – Total Fat 2 g – Saturated Fat 0 g – Cholesterol 0 mg – Sodium 55 mg – Total Carbohydrate 12 g Dietary Fibre 3 g – Sugars 7 g – Protein 2 g – Calcium 2% DV

Best Baked Beans

450 g (16 oz) canned butter beans
55 g (2 oz) frozen sweetcorn
2 chopped tomatoes
55 g (2 oz) Cheddar cheese, grated
Salt and pepper to taste

Preheat the oven to 180°C/350°F/gas mark 4. Combine
all ingredients and bake for 30 minutes. Makes 4 servings.

NUTRITION FACTS

Amount Per Serving: Calories 230 – Calories from Fat 50 – Total Fat 5 g – Saturated
Fat 3 g – Cholesterol 15 mg – Sodium 95 mg – Total Carbohydrate 32 g
Dietary Fibre 10 g – Sugars 2 g – Protein 14 g – Calcium 15% DV

Broccoli and Cauliflower in Lime Dressing

1 tablespoon low-sodium soya sauce
2 teaspoons raw honey
3 tablespoons fresh lime juice
75 g (2¾ oz) broccoli florets
100 g (3½ oz) cauliflower florets
Salt and pepper to taste
Red pepper flakes (optional)

Mix soya sauce, honey and lime juice. Set aside.

Boil broccoli and cauliflower for about 5 minutes, until they are tender yet firm. Drain and toss immediately with soya sauce–lime mixture. Season with salt and pepper to taste. Sprinkle with red pepper flakes if desired. Makes 4 servings.

NUTRITION FACTS

Amount Per Serving: Calories 30 – Calories from Fat 0 – Total Fat 0 g – Saturated Fat 0 g – Cholesterol 0 mg – Sodium 170 mg – Total Carbohydrate 7 g Dietary Fibre 1 g – Sugars 4 g – Protein 2 g – Calcium 2% DV

Cruciferous Couscous

90 g (3¼ oz) broccoli, chopped
50 g (1¾ oz) fresh spinach
90 g (3¼ oz) cauliflower, chopped
2 tomatoes, cubed
2 tablespoons minced garlic
2 tablespoons extra-virgin olive oil
750 ml (1¾ pint) water
350 g (12 oz) couscous
2 tablespoons balsamic vinegar
Salt and pepper to taste

Preheat oven to 180°C/350°F/gas mark 4. Mix broccoli, spinach, cauliflower and tomatoes with garlic and 1 tablespoon of olive oil and place on a baking sheet. Bake for 15–20 minutes, until tender. In a pot, bring water and remaining tablespoon of olive oil to the boil, add couscous and return to a boil, then remove from heat and let stand for 5 minutes. Fluff with a fork and let cool. Place couscous on a plate and top with roasted vegetables. Drizzle with balsamic vinegar before serving. Makes 8 servings.

NUTRITION FACTS

Amount Per Serving: Calories 220 – Calories from Fat 35 – Total Fat 4 g – Saturated Fat 0.5 g – Cholesterol 0 mg – Sodium 20 mg – Total Carbohydrate 38 g
Dietary Fibre 3 g – Sugars 2 g – Protein 6 g – Calcium 4% DV

Dressed-Up Asparagus

450 g (16 oz) fresh asparagus
2 tablespoons extra-virgin olive oil
2 teaspoons lemon juice
Salt and pepper to taste
1½ tablespoons finely chopped almonds
1 tablespoon toasted flaxseed

Wash asparagus and trim ends. Steam for 3–5 minutes, until bright green and tender but crisp. While asparagus is steaming, mix together olive oil, lemon juice, salt and pepper. In a separate bowl, mix the almonds and flaxseed. Drain asparagus and arrange on a serving platter. Drizzle with olive oil–lemon juice mixture and then sprinkle with nut-seed mix. Serve immediately. Makes 4 servings.

NUTRITION FACTS

Amount Per Serving: Calories 120 – Calories from Fat 80 – Total Fat 9 g – Saturated Fat 1 g – Cholesterol 0 mg – Sodium 0 mg – Total Carbohydrate 6 g – Dietary Fibre 3 g Sugars 3 g – Protein 3 g – Calcium 4% DV

Easy Pickled Beetroot

1.7 kg (3 lb 12 oz) cooked and peeled fresh
   beetroot
50 g (1¾ oz) xylitol (natural sugar substitute)
225 ml (8 fl oz) cider vinegar
125 ml (4 fl oz) orange juice

Drain beetroot. Mix sugar substitute, vinegar and orange
juice. Pour over beetroot and refrigerate overnight. Makes
8–10 servings.

NUTRITION FACTS

Amount Per Serving: Calories 60 – Calories from Fat 0 – Total Fat 0 g – Saturated
Fat 0 g – Cholesterol 0 mg – Sodium 95 mg – Total Carbohydrate 13 g
Dietary Fibre 2 g – Sugars 10 g – Protein 2 g – Calcium 2% DV

Green and Yellow Veggie Hash

2 small acorn squash, diced
2 carrots, grated
½ green apple, diced
1 shallot, finely chopped
3 tablespoons extra-virgin olive oil
45 g (1½ oz) greens (kale, spinach or turnip,
    spring or mustard greens), cleaned, washed
    and shredded
1 tablespoon minced garlic
4 sprigs fresh sage
Salt and pepper to taste

Sauté the squash, carrots, green apple and shallots in olive oil until tender. Mix in the greens, garlic, sage, salt, and pepper and continue cooking for 5 more minutes. Makes 6 servings.

NUTRITION FACTS

Amount Per Serving: Calories 140 – Calories from Fat 70 – Total Fat 7 g – Saturated Fat 1 g – Cholesterol 0 mg – Sodium 25 mg – Total Carbohydrate 20 g Dietary Fibre 3 g – Sugars 5 g – Protein 2 g – Calcium 6% DV

Asparagus with Sesame Seeds

4 tablespoons extra-virgin olive oil
450 g (16 oz) fresh asparagus, trimmed and
  peeled
1 teaspoon salt
1 tablespoon sesame seeds

Drizzle the olive oil over the asparagus and turn spears until they are coated. Sprinkle with salt. Grill asparagus for 5 minutes under a hot grill or on a hot barbecue, turning each minute or so. Remove and toss with sesame seeds. Makes 4 servings.

NUTRITION FACTS

Amount Per Serving: Calories 90 – Calories from Fat 70 – Total Fat 8 g – Saturated Fat 1 g – Cholesterol 0 mg – Sodium 0 mg – Total Carbohydrate 5 g – Dietary Fibre 3 g Sugars 2 g – Protein 3 g – Calcium 4% DV

Indian-Style Brussels Sprouts

2 tablespoons extra-virgin olive oil

1 teaspoon black or brown mustard seeds

2 teaspoons grated fresh ginger

1 teaspoon ground coriander

½ teaspoon turmeric

½ teaspoon ground cardamom

⅛ teaspoon cayenne pepper

12 Brussels sprouts, cut in half

125 ml (4 fl oz) unsweetened organic apple juice

2 tablespoons fresh lemon juice

Salt and pepper to taste

Heat the olive oil in a frying pan or saucepan. Add the mustard seeds and cook until they begin to pop. Stir in ginger, coriander, turmeric, cardamom, cayenne and Brussels sprouts. Pour in the apple and lemon juices, add salt and pepper, then cover and simmer until tender, about 5 minutes. Makes 6 servings.

NUTRITION FACTS

Amount Per Serving: Calories 90 – Calories from Fat 45 – Total Fat 5 g – Saturated Fat 0.5 g – Cholesterol 0 mg – Sodium 20 mg – Total Carbohydrate 10 g Dietary Fibre 3 g – Sugars 4 g – Protein 3 g – Calcium 4% DV

Kale and Sauerkraut

1 bunch kale
1 can sauerkraut, drained

Steam kale leaves until tender but still green. Stir in one can
of sauerkraut before serving.

NUTRITION FACTS

Amount Per Serving: Calories 30 – Calories from Fat 5 – Total Fat 0 g – Saturated Fat
0 g – Cholesterol 0 mg – Sodium 480 mg – Total Carbohydrate 7 g
Dietary Fibre 3 g – Sugars 1 g – Protein 2 g – Calcium 8% DV

Lemon-Curry Cauliflower and Kale

1 teaspoon curry powder
2 teaspoons lemon zest
3 tablespoons lemon juice
1 bunch kale
1 head cauliflower
Salt and pepper to taste

Mix curry powder, lemon zest and lemon juice. Set aside. Boil kale and cauliflower in a large pot of water with salt and pepper for 4–5 minutes, until tender. Drain and toss with lemon juice mixture. Makes 4 servings.

NUTRITION FACTS

Amount Per Serving: Calories 70 – Calories from Fat 5 – Total Fat 0.5 g – Saturated Fat 0 g – Cholesterol 0 mg – Sodium 70 mg – Total Carbohydrate 15 g Dietary Fibre 5 g – Sugars 4 g – Protein 5 g – Calcium 10% DV

Marinated Broccoli, Cucumber and Tomato Salad

1 head of broccoli
600 g (1 lb 5 oz) cucumbers
150 g (5½ oz) cherry tomatoes, halved
4 tablespoons extra-virgin olive oil
2 tablespoons lemon juice
175 ml (6 fl oz) cider vinegar
3 tablespoons parsley, minced
Salt and pepper to taste
55 g (2 oz) low-fat feta cheese
Fresh spinach

Cut the broccoli into florets and steam for 3 minutes; let cool. Chop the cucumber into bite-sized pieces, toss with cherry tomatoes and then add the cooled broccoli. In a small bowl, mix olive oil, lemon juice, vinegar, parsley, salt and pepper. Pour the mixture over the vegetables. Place in refrigerator and chill overnight. Toss with feta cheese right before serving on a bed of spinach. Makes 8 servings.

NUTRITION FACTS

Amount Per Serving: Calories 110 – Calories from Fat 70 – Total Fat 8 g – Saturated Fat 1.5 g – Cholesterol 0 mg – Sodium 115 mg – Total Carbohydrate 6 g Dietary Fibre 2 g – Sugars 3 g – Protein 4 g – Calcium 6% DV

Mashed Cauliflower

675 g (1 lb 8 oz) cauliflower
Salt and pepper to taste
60 ml (2 fl oz) skimmed milk
15 g (½ oz) instant low-carb mashed potatoes
1 teaspoon garlic paste or garlic powder
2 rashers cooked turkey bacon, crumbled

Cut cauliflower into florets and steam with salt and pepper until very tender. Place in blender and add all ingredients except turkey bacon. Blend until smooth. Return to pot to reheat if necessary. Garnish with crumbled turkey bacon. Makes 4 servings.

NUTRITION FACTS

Amount Per Serving: Calories 110 – Calories from Fat 40 – Total Fat 4.5 g
Saturated Fat 1.5 g – Cholesterol 15 mg – Sodium 380 mg – Total Carbohydrate 13 g
Dietary Fibre 4 g – Sugars 4 g – Protein 8 g – Calcium 6% DV

Roasted Beetroot

8 beetroot, peeled and quartered
3 tablespoons extra-virgin olive oil
1 teaspoon salt
1 teaspoon pepper

Preheat oven to 220°C/425°F/gas mark 7. Place beetroot in a large baking tin and toss with oil, salt and pepper. Bake for 1 hour and 30 minutes. Makes 6 servings.

NUTRITION FACTS

Amount Per Serving: Calories 110 – Calories from Fat 60 – Total Fat 7 g
Saturated Fat 1 g – Cholesterol 0 mg – Sodium 480 mg – Total Carbohydrate 11 g
Dietary Fibre 3 g – Sugars 7 g – Protein 2 g – Calcium 2% DV

Swede and Nutmeg

4 large swede
¼ teaspoon salt
Water
1 tablespoon extra-virgin olive oil
Black pepper
Dash of nutmeg

Peel swede with a vegetable peeler and cut into chunks. Put them in a saucepan, add the salt and cover with water. Bring to the boil. Turn heat down to medium and cook 12–15 minutes, or until fork tender. Drain, but save the cooking liquid.

Using a potato masher, coarsely mash the swede in the saucepan, adding the cooking liquid as needed for moisture. Add olive oil, more salt if necessary and pepper to taste. Transfer to a serving bowl and garnish with a dash of nutmeg. Makes 6 servings.

NUTRITION FACTS

Amount Per Serving: Calories 110 – Calories from Fat 25 – Total Fat 3 g – Saturated Fat 0 g – Cholesterol 0 mg – Sodium 150 mg – Total Carbohydrate 21 g Dietary Fibre 6 g – Sugars 14 g – Protein 3 g – Calcium 10% DV

Simple Greens and Garlic

Note: This recipe works well for kale, spinach, turnip greens, spring greens or rocket.

> 3 tablespoons extra-virgin olive oil
> 1 onion, chopped
> 3 cloves garlic, minced
> 900 g (2 lb) greens, washed, dried and
>   shredded
> Salt and pepper

Heat olive oil over medium-high heat in a large frying pan. Add onion and garlic; cook and stir until soft. Stir in greens and cook until wilted. Salt and pepper to taste. Serve hot or warm. Makes 4 servings.

NUTRITION FACTS

Amount Per Serving: Calories 180 – Calories from Fat 100 – Total Fat 11 g
Saturated Fat 1.5 g – Cholesterol 0 mg – Sodium 45 mg – Total Carbohydrate 16 g
Dietary Fibre 9 g – Sugars 2 g – Protein 6 g – Calcium 35% DV

Broccoli or Asparagus with Sesame Seeds

2 large stalks fresh broccoli or
   12–14 asparagus spears
2 tablespoons extra-virgin olive oil
2 tablespoons sesame seeds
2 or 3 cloves garlic, peeled and sliced
Salt and pepper to taste

Wash broccoli and cut the florets into medium to large pieces. Peel the tough outer layer from the stems and slice the inner tender, juicy portion in half. Or, if using asparagus, wash the spears and trim off the ends. In a large frying pan with a lid, heat the oil over high heat. Add sesame seeds and sauté, stirring until lightly toasted; be careful not to over-cook, because they burn quickly. Also, keep the lid handy because the sesame seeds might start to pop. Add the broccoli (or asparagus) and garlic, and stir for a few seconds. Add salt and pepper to taste, and stir. Cover the frying pan and remove from heat; let sit about 15 minutes. The broccoli (or asparagus) will retain its colour and be tender and crisp. Makes 6 servings.

NUTRITION FACTS

Amount Per Serving: Calories 70 – Calories from Fat 50 – Total Fat 6 g – Saturated Fat 1 g – Cholesterol 0 mg – Sodium 0 mg – Total Carbohydrate 3 g – Dietary Fibre 1 g Sugars 1 g – Protein 1 g – Calcium 4% DV

Spinach and Feta Brown Rice

200 g (7 oz) brown rice
35 g (1¾ oz) fresh spinach leaves
2 teaspoons minced garlic
55 g (2 oz) low-fat feta cheese
Salt and pepper to taste

Cook the brown rice according to directions on the packet, or bring to the boil 2 parts water to 1 part rice in a medium-sized pot, then cook on low for 30–45 minutes until the rice is soft. Before serving, add the spinach and garlic, stirring until the spinach wilts. Put on a plate and garnish with feta cheese. Makes 6 servings.

NUTRITION FACTS

Amount Per Serving: Calories 120 – Calories from Fat 15 – Total Fat 1.5 g
Saturated Fat 0.5 g – Cholesterol 0 mg – Sodium 70 mg – Total Carbohydrate 24 g
Dietary Fibre 1 g – Sugars 0 g – Protein 4 g – Calcium 2% DV

SALADS, SALAD DRESSINGS AND SNACKS

Banana in Bark

1 tablespoon ground almonds
1 tablespoon ground or milled flaxseed
1 whole banana

Mix almonds and flaxseeds on a large plate. Peel banana and roll in mixture until fully covered. Either eat immediately or place on waxed paper and put in refrigerator to chill before eating. Makes 1 serving.

NUTRITION FACTS

Amount Per Serving: Calories 200 – Calories from Fat 70 – Total Fat 7 g
Saturated Fat 0.5 g Cholesterol 0 mg – Sodium 0 mg – Total Carbohydrate 36 g
Dietary Fibre 6 g – Sugars 20 g – Protein 4 g Calcium 4% DV

Beetroot and Orange Salad

1 jar pickled beetroot
2 cans mandarin oranges in water, or 2 tangerines, peeled, sectioned and seeded
125 ml (4 fl oz) orange juice
35 g (1¾ oz) fresh spinach
25 g (1 oz) flaked almonds

Toss beetroot and mandarin orange or tangerine sections in orange juice. Chill for at least 1 hour. Serve on bed of spinach. Garnish with flaked almonds. Makes 4 servings.

NUTRITION FACTS

Amount Per Serving: Calories 150 – Calories from Fat 30 – Total Fat 3.5 g
Saturated Fat 0 g – Cholesterol 0 mg – Sodium 80 mg – Total Carbohydrate 28 g
Dietary Fibre 4 g – Sugars 22 g – Protein 4 g – Calcium 6% DV

Cabbage-Apple Salad

90 g (3¼ oz) cabbage, shredded
175 g (7 oz) apple, diced
125 g (4½ oz) celery, chopped
70 g (2½ oz) natural low-fat yoghurt
2 tablespoons flaxseed

Mix all ingredients in a large bowl. Toss, chill and serve.
Makes 6 servings.

NUTRITION FACTS
Amount Per Serving: Calories 45 – Calories from Fat 15 – Total Fat 2 g
Saturated Fat 0 g – Cholesterol 0 mg – Sodium 25 mg – Total Carbohydrate 7 g
Dietary Fibre 2 g – Sugars 4 g – Protein 2 g – Calcium 4% DV

Carrot and Orange Salad

115 g (4 oz) carrots, grated
½ teaspoon lemon juice
2 tablespoons frozen orange
    juice concentrate
1 tablespoon natural low-fat yoghurt
450 g (16 oz) low-fat cottage cheese
280 g (10 oz) canned mandarin oranges packed
    in water (not syrup), drained
Fresh spinach

Mix all ingredients in a large bowl except for half of the mandarin oranges and spinach. Place salad on a bed of spinach for each serving. Garnish each serving with the remaining mandarin oranges. Makes 6 servings.

NUTRITION FACTS

Amount Per Serving: Calories 90 – Calories from Fat 10 – Total Fat 1 g
Saturated Fat 0.5 g – Cholesterol 5 mg – Sodium 350 mg – Total Carbohydrate 11 g
Dietary Fibre 2 g – Sugars 8 g – Protein 11 g – Calcium 10% DV

Chicken and Cold Rice Salad

400 g (14 oz) cooked brown rice (you may use
    whole-grain quick-cooking brown rice)
350 g (12 oz) cooked chicken, cubed
70 g (2½ oz) broccoli florets, steamed al dente
55 g (2 oz) flaked almonds
2 tablespoons minced parsley
300 g (10½ oz) natural low-fat yoghurt
Spinach
4 tangerines

Toss everything together in a large bowl except the
spinach and tangerines. Chill for at least 2 hours. Serve
on a bed of spinach and surround with tangerine slices.
Makes 10 servings.

NUTRITION FACTS

Amount Per Serving: Calories 170 – Calories from Fat 40 – Total Fat 4.5 g – Saturated
Fat 1 g – Cholesterol 30 mg – Sodium 70 mg – Total Carbohydrate 18 g
Dietary Fibre 3 g – Sugars 6 g – Protein 15 g – Calcium 10% DV

Celebration Salsa

4 ripe tomatoes, diced
4 spring onions, chopped
1 large cucumber, minced
1 large orange, sectioned, seeded and cut into
    small pieces
1 tablespoon fresh coriander, minced
2 tablespoons lemon juice
Salt to taste

Combine all ingredients in a large bowl. Refrigerate for at least 1 hour before serving to allow flavours to blend. This will keep in the refrigerator for 2–3 days. Makes 6 servings.

NUTRITION FACTS

Amount Per Serving: Calories 35 – Calories from Fat 5 – Total Fat 0 g
Saturated Fat 0 g – Cholesterol 0 mg – Sodium 10 mg – Total Carbohydrate 8 g
Dietary Fibre 2 g – Sugars 5 g – Protein 1 g – Calcium 4% DV

Creamy Coleslaw

360 g (12½ oz) cabbage, shredded
115 g (4 oz) carrots, grated
450 g (16 oz) natural low-fat yoghurt
1½ tablespoons finely chopped celery
1 teaspoon grated onion
3 tablespoons white vinegar
1 tablespoon raw honey
¾ teaspoon salt
Dash of pepper

Mix all ingredients in a large bowl and toss well.
Refrigerate for at least 2 hours before serving. Makes 10
servings.

NUTRITION FACTS

Amount Per Serving: Calories 40 – Calories from Fat 5 – Total Fat 0.5 g – Total
Carbohydrate 7 g – Dietary Fibre 1 g – Sugars 6 g – Protein 2 g – Calcium 8% DV

Cucumber and Yoghurt Dressing

1 large cucumber
300 g (10½ oz) natural low-fat yoghurt
1 tablespoon extra-virgin olive oil
½ teaspoon salt
½ teaspoon dill

Combine all ingredients in a blender and blend well.
Refrigerate for at least 1 hour, then serve. This will keep in
the refrigerator for 2 days. Makes 6 servings.

NUTRITION FACTS

Amount Per Serving: Calories 50 – Calories from Fat 25 – Total Fat 3 g – Saturated
Fat 0.5 g – Cholesterol 0 mg – Sodium 220 mg – Total Carbohydrate 4 g – Dietary
Fibre 0 g – Sugars 4 g – Protein 2 g – Calcium 8% DV

Favourite Chicken Salad

4 x 115 g (4 oz) chicken breasts, boiled and
  diced
4 hard-boiled eggs, sliced
115 g (4 oz) celery, sliced
1 medium apple, chopped
150 g (5½ oz) natural low-fat yoghurt
2 tablespoons lemon juice
1 teaspoon salt
1 teaspoon pepper
Fresh spinach
70 g (2½ oz) almonds, finely chopped

Combine all ingredients except almonds. Place in refrigerator for at least 4 hours. Serve over fresh spinach and top with chopped almonds. Makes 8 servings.

NUTRITION FACTS

Amount Per Serving: Calories 190 – Calories from Fat 70 – Total Fat 8 g – Saturated
Fat 2 g – Cholesterol 155 mg – Sodium 390 mg – Total Carbohydrate 6 g
Dietary Fibre 2 g – Sugars 4 g – Protein 23 g – Calcium 8% DV

Flaxseed and Fruit Smoothie

225 ml (8 fl oz) skimmed milk
225 g (8 oz) frozen berries
1 banana
300 g (10½ oz) natural low-fat yoghurt
1 tablespoon flaxseed oil
1 tablespoon ground flaxseed

Combine all ingredients except flaxseed in blender. Blend well. Pour into large glass and stir in flaxseed. Makes 1 serving.

NUTRITION FACTS

Amount Per Serving: Calories 580 – Calories from Fat 200 – Total Fat 23 g –
Saturated Fat 4 g – Cholesterol 20 mg – Sodium 310 mg – Total Carbohydrate 78 g
Dietary Fibre 7 g – Sugars 58 g – Protein 25 g – Calcium 70% DV

Ginger-Lime Dressing

1 cup low-sodium soya sauce
2 tablespoons minced garlic
2 tablespoons grated fresh ginger
2 teaspoons sesame oil
90 ml (3 fl oz) fresh lime juice
60 ml (2 fl oz) rice vinegar

Place all ingredients in blender. Blend until well mixed. Chill for at least 1 hour, then serve. Makes 6 servings.

NUTRITION FACTS

Amount Per Serving: Calories 50 – Calories from Fat 15 – Total Fat 1.5 g – Saturated Fat 0 g – Cholesterol 0 mg – Sodium 1600 mg – Total Carbohydrate 7 g Dietary Fibre 1 g – Sugars 1 g – Protein 3 g – Calcium 2% DV

Grapefruit and Avocado Salad

2 whole Ruby Red grapefruits
1 medium ripe avocado
3 tablespoons orange juice
2 tablespoons natural low-fat yoghurt
1 teaspoon raw honey
1 teaspoon poppy seeds
Fresh spinach

Peel, section and deseed grapefruit. Peel avocado and slice lengthways. Mix orange juice, yoghurt and honey, whisking until well blended. Stir in poppy seeds. Arrange grapefruit and avocado together on bed of spinach. Drizzle with orange–poppy seed dressing. Makes 4 servings.

NUTRITION FACTS

Amount Per Serving: Calories 130 – Calories from Fat 60 – Total Fat 6 g – Saturated Fat 1 g – Cholesterol 0 mg – Sodium 30 mg – Total Carbohydrate 19 g Dietary Fibre 3 g – Sugars 3 g – Protein 3 g – Calcium 6% DV

Grated Beetroot Salad

2 tablespoons lemon juice
¾ cup orange juice
900 g (2 lb) fresh beetroot, peeled and grated
Salt and pepper to taste
20 g (¾ oz) fresh parsley, chopped

Add lemon juice to orange juice and stir. Toss in grated beetroot. Add salt and pepper. Chill at least 1 hour and toss in parsley before serving. Makes 8 servings.

NUTRITION FACTS

Amount Per Serving: Calories 60 – Calories from Fat 0 – Total Fat 0 g – Saturated Fat 0 g – Cholesterol 0 mg – Sodium 90 mg – Total Carbohydrate 14 g Dietary Fibre 2 g – Sugars 11 g – Protein 2 g – Calcium 2% – DV

Marinated Cucumber, Radish and Onion Salad

125 ml (4 fl oz) rice wine vinegar
60 ml (2 fl oz) extra-virgin olive oil
1 tablespoon chopped fresh dill or
    1 teaspoon dried dill
1 large cucumber, sliced thin
55 g (2 oz) radishes, sliced
1 medium red onion, sliced thin

Mix vinegar, olive oil and dill in a large bowl. Add cucumber, radishes and onion. Toss to coat. Refrigerate at least 3 hours, stirring at least once an hour to allow flavours to meld. Makes 8 servings.

NUTRITION FACTS

Amount Per Serving: Calories 80 – Calories from Fat 60 – Total Fat 7 g – Saturated Fat 1 g – Cholesterol 0 mg – Sodium 0 mg – Total Carbohydrate 4 g Dietary Fibre 1 g – Sugars 2 g – Protein 0 g – Calcium 2% DV

Not Your Ordinary Tuna Salad

350 g (12 oz) canned white albacore tuna in
   water
1 red pepper, chopped fine
1 yellow pepper, chopped fine
1 small green apple, grated
30 g (1 oz) fresh cabbage, shredded
2 tablespoons natural low-fat yoghurt
½ teaspoon lemon juice
½ teaspoon rice wine vinegar
Salt and pepper to taste

Mix all ingredients together in a large bowl. Chill for at least
1 hour before serving. Makes 4 servings.

NUTRITION FACTS

Amount Per Serving: Calories 70 – Calories from Fat 15 – Total Fat 1.5 g – Saturated
Fat 0 g – Cholesterol 20 mg – Sodium 170 mg – Total Carbohydrate 4 g
Dietary Fibre 1 g – Sugars 3 g – Protein 11 g – Calcium 2% DV

Sauerkraut Salad

450 g (16 oz) canned sauerkraut
680 g (1 lb 8 oz) onion, chopped
190 g (6½ oz) pimento, sliced
475 g (1 lb 1 oz) celery, chopped
175 g (6 oz) broccoli, chopped
125 ml (4 fl oz) white vinegar
Salt and pepper to taste

Toss all ingredients together in a very large bowl and refrigerate overnight. This will keep in the refrigerator for up to a week. Makes 12 servings.

NUTRITION FACTS

Amount Per Serving: Calories 40 – Calories from Fat 0 – Total Fat 0 g – Saturated Fat 0 g – Cholesterol 0 mg – Sodium 290 mg – Total Carbohydrate 9 g Dietary Fibre 3 g – Sugars 4 g – Protein 2 g – Calcium 4% DV

Simple Cheese on Toast

Organic non-stick cooking spray
6 slices wholemeal bread
Extra-virgin olive oil
2 tomatoes, sliced
3 tablespoons grated Cheddar cheese
3 tablespoons grated skimmed milk mozzarella
 cheese

Preheat the grill. Arrange bread on flat baking sheet that you have sprayed with organic non-stick baking spray. Brush bread tops with olive oil. Toast under the grill for a few minutes or until bread is firm and crisp to the touch. Remove and top each piece of bread with a slice of tomato; sprinkle with cheese. Return bread to the grill and heat until cheese melts and is bubbly, usually less than 3 minutes. Makes 6 servings.

NUTRITION FACTS

Amount Per Serving: Calories 110 – Calories from Fat 30 – Total Fat 3.5 g
Saturated Fat 1.5 g – Cholesterol 5 mg – Sodium 180 mg – Total Carbohydrate 14 g
Dietary Fibre 2 g – Sugars 4 g – Protein 6 g – Calcium 6% DV

Spinach Salad with Beetroot in Cottage Cheese

4 medium beetroot
60 ml (2 fl oz) extra-virgin olive oil
3 tablespoons lemon juice
½ teaspoon raw honey
¼ teaspoon dry mustard
Salt and pepper to taste
115 g (4 oz) low-fat cottage cheese
2 tablespoons milled flaxseed
90 g (3¼ oz) fresh spinach

Boil beetroot until tender and let cool. While beetroot are cooling, mix olive oil, lemon juice, raw honey, dry mustard and salt and pepper. Peel and slice beetroot into strips, then mix with cottage cheese and flaxseed. Place on bed of spinach. Drizzle the salad with the dressing mixture. Makes 4 servings.

NUTRITION FACTS

Amount Per Serving: Calories 210 – Calories from Fat 150 – Total Fat 16 g
Saturated Fat 2.5 g – Cholesterol 0 mg – Sodium 190 mg – Total Carbohydrate 12 g
Dietary Fibre 4 g – Sugars 7 g – Protein 6 g – Calcium 6% DV

Yoghurt and Fruit Parfait

30 g (1 oz) ground almonds
2 tablespoons ground or milled flaxseed
300 g (10½ oz) natural low-fat yoghurt
115 g (4 oz) berries
Raw honey (optional)

In small bowl, mix almonds with flaxseed. In parfait glass, alternately layer yoghurt, berries and almond-flaxseed mixture. If desired, drizzle a small amount of honey on top. Makes 1 serving.

NUTRITION FACTS

Amount Per Serving: Calories 480 – Calories from Fat 240 – Total Fat 27 g
Saturated Fat 4.5 g – Cholesterol 15 mg – Sodium 180 mg – Total Carbohydrate 47 g
Dietary Fibre 8 g – Sugars 25 g – Protein 23 g – Calcium 60% DV

APPENDIX A

Journal and Food Diary

Many of the people who have been successful on the plan report that they made the best progress when they monitored themselves by writing things down. The following can be used as your daily tracking tool. Make thirty copies, one for each day of the month, and fill in every day.

Date: _____

Weight: _____

Waistline measurement
(first week of each month only): _____

A. Circle the reply that best fits for each of the following categories.
   1. Sleep:
      • a full eight hours

- sporadically waking up through the night with hot flushes
- not sleeping at all

2. Energy:
   - rested and ready to go
   - sluggish and slow
   - fatigued; wish I could go back to bed

3. Mood:
   - extremely upbeat
   - positive
   - indifferent
   - irritable and moody
   - depressed

4. Libido, sex drive:
   - always strong
   - very high right now
   - not great now but never good in the morning
   - neutral or indifferent
   - very low
   - comatose

5. Body image:
   - feel good about my body size and shape
   - feel positive about some weight loss and change in body shape
   - feel just okay
   - feel frustrated

B. Check the symptoms of hormone imbalance that you are experiencing today.
   1. Women:
      ❏ Weight gain ❏ Mood swings ❏ Hot flushes

❑ Night sweats ❑ Fatigue ❑ Headaches
❑ Depression ❑ Anxiety ❑ Nervousness
❑ Irritability ❑ Teariness ❑ Memory lapse
❑ Premature ageing ❑ Vaginal dryness
❑ Heavy menses ❑ Bleeding changes
❑ Incontinence ❑ Fibrocystic breasts
❑ Decreased sex drive ❑ Tender breasts
❑ Osteoporosis ❑ Water retention

2. Premenopausal or perimenopausal women:
   • My last menstrual cycle started on _____ (date).
   • I am currently menstruating; this is the _____ day
     of my cycle.

3. Men:
   ❑ Weight gain ❑ Burned-out feeling
   ❑ Abdominal fat ❑ Prostate problems
   ❑ Decreased mental clarity ❑ Decreased sex drive
   ❑ Increased urinary urge ❑ Decreased strength
   ❑ Decreased stamina ❑ Difficulty sleeping
   ❑ Decreased urine flow ❑ Irritability
   ❑ Depression ❑ Erectile dysfunction
   ❑ Hot flushes ❑ Night sweats ❑ Poor concentration

C. Stress level
   1. On a scale of 0–10 (0 = no stress; 10 = high stress), my
      stress level is _____.

D. Exercise
   1. Last week I exercised _____ times per week for an
      average of _____ minutes each time.
   2. Describe the activity or activities: _____
      _____

E. Outlook

1. In addition to being grateful for making progress towards losing my unwanted belly fat, I am thankful for (list three things): _____

_____

_____

Your Belly Flat Food Diary

Most nutritionists and dietitians agree that keeping a food diary is critical to weight loss success. Keeping a thirty-day food diary will help you make hormone-healthy eating an easy habit to keep. It will also help you better identify when, where, how and with whom all your good intentions go by the wayside to the detriment of your waist size.

Here are a three helpful hints:

• **Write everything down.**

Keep your diary with you all day. Write down every mouthful, even chewing gum.

• **Tell the truth.**

The only thing you have to gain by cheating on these forms is more weight.

• **Do it now.**

Don't depend on your memory at the end of the day. Record everything you eat and drink as soon as it is consumed.

Daily Food Diary

Date:_____

	Time	What Did You Eat? Drink?	How Much?	Where?	With Whom?	What Were You Doing?	What Was Your Mood?
Breakfast							
Snack							
Lunch							
Snack							
Dinner							

Belly-Blasting Food Checklist

Food Group	Recommended Servings/Day	# of Servings You Had
Cruciferous Vegetables	2–3	
Citrus Fruit	1	
Insoluble Fibre	2	
Lignans	2–3 tablespoons	
Protein	3	
Calcium	2	
Fruit (other than citrus)	1	
Water	8–10 glasses	

Don't Forget to Supplement Your Weight Loss Success

Supplement	Recommended Dosage	What You Took	What Time
Bio-Identical Progesterone Cream	• Women who are menstruating: twice daily from day 8–26 of your cycle • Women who are no longer menstruating or who are perimenopausal: twice daily for 25 days, then take 5 days off • Women also on bio-identical oestrogen: twice daily, every day • Men: twice daily for 25 days then 5 days off		
Calcium D-Glucarate	1,000 mg twice daily		
DIM	Women should take 200 mg per day; men 400 mg per day		
B-Complex Vitamin	1 per day		
Vitamin E	400 IU per day		
Calcium-Magnesium Supplement	1,500 mg of calcium and 750 mg of magnesium		
7-Keto DHEA	100 mg each morning		
Chitosan	750 mg to 1 g three times daily; take with meals		

How Did You Take Care of You Today? Did You . . .

Activity	Doing What?	What Time?	How Long?	With Whom?
Consciously Take Time To De-Stress				
Exercise				
Laugh				
Sleep				

APPENDIX B

How to Reduce the Oestrogens in Your Environment

The following list can help you to take action to reduce the effect of environmental oestrogens in your life:

- Because some plastics shed xenohormones when heated, assume that they all do, and protect yourself accordingly. Don't drink hot beverages from plastic cups and don't drink water from a plastic bottle that has been left in the sun or in a hot car.
- Don't microwave your food or drinks in plastic containers; avoid using cling film to cover food in the microwave.
- Get a good-quality water filter for your home. Drink and cook with filtered water.

- When possible, eat only organic, hormone-free meat and dairy products.
- Eat organic produce, which has not been sprayed with pesticides.
- Wash all produce to rid it of any type of chemical residue or pesticides.
- Throw away all pesticides, herbicides and fungicides.
- Never tent your house and fumigate it with pesticides.
- Research and use organic approaches and products for home gardening and pest control.
- Check product labels for the following chemicals: aliphatic hydrocarbons (n-hexane), halogenated hydrocarbons (carbon tetrachloride, trichlorethylene), alcohols (methanol, ethanol), cyclic hydrocarbons (cyclohexane), esters (ethyl acetate), ethers (ethyl ether), nitrohydrocarbons (ethyl nitrate), ketones (acetone, methylethylketone), glycols (ethylene glycol), aromatic hydrocarbons (benzene) and aldehydes (acetaldehyde). Do not buy products, or throw away those you already have, if these chemicals are present.
- Check your cosmetics for toxic ingredients and throw them away. Most health food stores now stock a variety of organic cosmetics and even natural hair dyes.
- Don't use fabric softeners.
- Exchange your perfumes and air fresheners for natural aromatic oils and fresh scents from your garden.
- Because most spermicidal products contain petrochemicals, avoid using lubricated condoms or vaginal gels.
- New homes or offices filled with new carpet, fibreboard,

new paint and glues can give off a wide variety of toxic fumes. Consider flushing the toxins out of the air with a portable air filter prior to moving in.

- Never use synthetic hormone replacement.
- Evaluate your options for birth control and, whenever possible, find an alternative to birth control pills. If your personal choice is to use birth control pills for contraception, use for the shortest term possible.

APPENDIX C

Resources

Please note: The contact information listed in this section is current as of the publication of this book and is specific to the US.

For UK readers, more information on natural progesterone, including details of how to obtain natural progesterone cream, can be found at: www.progesteronelink.com

Hormone saliva tests, plus a range of other tests, can be arranged by contacting Nature's Healing at:
Judy Evans, ND, Dip. Herb, MANP, MURHP
Naturopathic Practitioner and Medical Herbalist
Nature's Healing
Tel: 01935 474343
Email: info@natureshealing.org

Hormone Health

The Natural Hormone Institute of America
When Genie James and I co-founded The Natural Hormone Institute of America in 2003, we had two goals in mind. The

first was to create a vehicle to educate both the medical
community and healthcare consumers about the safety and
efficacy of bio-identical hormone therapies. Our second goal
was to make my over-the-counter bio-identical progesterone
cream and other products more widely available, committing
a percentage of website profits to support medical research in
the field of bio-identical hormone replacement.

To date, I have been overwhelmed by the positive response
of many of my physician peers, as well as interested and
educated healthcare consumers. I am grateful that The
Natural Hormone Institute of America is meeting a very real
need.

For more information regarding bio-identical hormone
replacement, to discuss scheduling a personal consultation or
to purchase the products recommended in this book, go to
my interactive website www.hormonewell.com, or contact
our office by telephone at 001-904-694-0039.

Over-the-Counter Progesterone Creams

You can purchase bio-identical progesterone creams in most
health food stores. The good news is that these creams are
available; the bad news is that some products are better than
others. The reason for this discrepancy: there is no regulatory
body that oversees the production or standardisation of product manufacturing for so-called 'natural' products. What this
means to the average consumer is that there is great variation
among the many OTC progesterone creams on the market
today.

While I cannot reveal the exact formula for my Natural

Balance Cream, I can outline some of the critical variables that define its excellence and efficacy:

- *Dr Randolph's Natural Balance Cream is a bio-identical formulation of progesterone.* This means that the molecules of progesterone suspended in the cream have exactly the same molecular structure as those produced by the human body. The body recognises, receives and utilises these molecules. The parent molecule for progesterone comes from a substance known as *diosgenin,* which is found in soya or Mexican wild yam. Many products on the market today containing soya or Mexican wild yam claim to be a 'natural progesterone'; however, until the diosgenin is converted from its original molecular structure, the body will not recognise it. Consequently, soya or Mexican wild yam in the raw state will not generate the same clinical response.
- *My Natural Balance Cream contains the maximum concentration of human-identical progesterone that can be mixed in an over-the-counter product.* Some creams have a small amount of progesterone in their mix, but not enough to generate a consistent and positive patient response.
- The progesterone I use in my formula meets the United States Pharmacopoeia gold standards for quality and purity. In addition, the lab I use to compound my cream operates under strict guidelines approved by the National Association of Compounding Pharmacists. This is *not* required by law, so not all product manufacturers go to the trouble or expense.
- *The progesterone molecule in my cream is encased within a liposomal delivery system.* This is critical because, as the

many layers of the oily globule of liposome melt away like a snowball, the hormones are dispersed continuously through the skin for up to twelve hours. This means that the underlying issue of hormonal imbalance is eliminated, hormonal balance is restored and my patients have continuous relief of their symptoms throughout the day. In contrast, many over-the-counter progesterone creams are not formulated for sustained release. All the progesterone in these creams is immediately absorbed through the skin, resulting in a quick spike in progesterone levels and a temporary versus constant relief of symptoms.

If you have any doubt or concerns regarding any bio-identical progesterone product, call the company and ask how many milligrams of progesterone per ounce the cream contains.

Testing Hormone Levels

If you have not found relief from your symptoms from using a progesterone cream, this can be regarded as a signal that your hormone levels have begun to fluctuate. At this time, a saliva test or capillary blood spot testing may be an appropriate next step to evaluate the current ratio of all three sex hormones.

On my website, I offer a viable option for those women or men who believe or have evidence that their hormone balance has shifted and requires treatment. You can go to www.hormonewell.com/hormoneconsultation.html to learn more about how you can obtain a comprehensive hormone level profile via a saliva test or schedule a one-on-one telephone consultation with me or one of my personally trained nurse practitioners.

ZRT Laboratory's state-of-the-art saliva and capillary blood spot testing technology allows for accurate measurement of a broad array of hormones and detection of existing hormone imbalance.

1. *Saliva Testing*

Convenient home collection, accurate and inexpensive, saliva testing provides a true picture of the bioavailable levels of steroid hormones.

2. *Capillary Blood Spot Testing*

Capillary blood spot testing offers an easy, finger-stick alternative to blood draws in the doctor's office.

3. *Combination Saliva and Capillary Blood Spot*

Combines both saliva and capillary blood spot test materials in an all-in-one test kit for easy home collection of the major hormone groups – reproductive, adrenal and thyroid – on the same day at the optimal time.

Dr David Zava, the founder of ZRT Laboratory, is also the co-author with John R Lee, MD, of *What Your Doctor May Not Tell You About Breast Cancer*.

To find out more information, contact:

ZRT Laboratory
8605 SW Creekside Place
Beaverton, OR 97008 US

Phone: 001-503-466-2445
Fax: 001-503-466-1636
24-Hour Hotline: 001-503-466-9166
Website: www.zrtlab.com

Locating a Doctor

There are two resources that I recommend if you are looking for a doctor in your area who is knowledgeable about bio-identical hormone replacement. The first is the Women In Balance website, www.womeninbalance.org. The second is your local compounding pharmacist. If you need help finding a compounding pharmacy in your area, contact one of the two organisations listed below.

The International Academy of Compounding Pharmacists (IACP)

P.O. Box 1365
Sugar Land, TX 77487 US
Phone: 001-281-933-8400
Fax: 001-281-495-0602
Website: www.iacprx.org

IACP was established in 1991 as Professionals and Patients for Customized Care (P2C2). In 1996, P2C2 changed its name to IACP in an effort to broaden its scope and recognise changes in the profession. Today, the IACP has more than 1,800 members internationally, serving pharmacists, physicians, students and patients.

Professional Compounding Centers of America (PCCA)
9901 South Wilcrest Drive
Houston, TX 77099 US
Phone: 001-877-798-3224
Fax: 001-877-765-1422
Website: www.pccarx.com

PCCA provides independent pharmacists with a complete support system from compounding unique dosage forms. Founded in 1981, PCCA has more than 3,000 pharmacist members located throughout the United States, Canada, Australia, Europe and New Zealand. On average, PCCA's consulting department answers more than 500 calls per day, providing members with comprehensive technical support.

'Belly Flat' Foods and Products

Organic Foods

Supermarkets

Because of growing consumer demand, almost every supermarket around the world stocks some organic foods. Still, my hat is off to two companies that over the last decade have taken the lead. They are:

Whole Foods: Founded in 1980 as one small store in Austin, Texas, Whole Foods is now the world's leading retailer of natural and organic foods, with 197 stores in North America and the United Kingdom. To find a Whole Foods near you, go to www.wholefoodsmarket.com.

Wild Oats: In July 2007 it was announced that Wild Oats, another pioneer, would merge with Whole Foods. Prior to the merger, Wild Oats operated 110 natural foods stores in 24 states and British Columbia, Canada. The Company's markets also include: Wild Oats Marketplace, Henry's Farmers Market, Sun Harvest and Capers Community Markets. At the time of this printing, Wild Oats website was still operational: www.wildoats.com.

Websites

Many people initially complain that buying organic is too expensive. Yes, organic foods can be pricey if you just shop in your supermarket, but you probably have a lot more choices for organic food in your community than you realise. All it takes is a little research to find out.

To find a source of organic foods near you or to order online, check out the following websites: www.organicfood.com, www.organicconsumer.org, www.eatwell.com and www. diamondorganics.com. Also, local farmer's markets can be a great source for organic foods, often at lower prices than you will pay in the supermarket or health food store.

Favourite Brands

Vitamins and Supplements

When I opened my first Natural Medicine Store, I stocked the shelves with natural products from a variety of manufacturers. It was not long before the difference in my patients' and customers' responses signalled to me that not all product manufacturers could be trusted. According to a recent survey of nearly 1,000 supplements conducted by ConsumerLab.com, a product-certification company, one out of four supplements has quality problems, such as contamination or a failure to include an ingredient listed on the label.

As I became aware of the discrepancy between manufacturers, I drew on my professional training and experience as a compounding pharmacist to establish criteria that would insure that any product in my shop and on my website was safe and effective.

My criterion for my private-label products was and is simple yet non-negotiable: **quality and truth in labelling**. This means that for my own private-labelled line, as well as other natural health product lines that I carry, I require stringent guidelines for their manufacturing process. These guidelines include:

- Raw materials testing
- Potency testing
- Product traceability
- Purity testing
- Product freshness
- Microbiology testing

The bottom line is truth in packaging. People have the right to know what they are putting in their bodies and they deserve to get the amount of active ingredient they are paying for.

To order Dr Randolph's products online, go to www. hormonewell.com/shop_online.htm.

Life Extension is a highly reputable source for vitamins and supplements. This company's manufacturing standards ensure exceptional purity and quality. For Life Extension members purchasing products, the company provides access to a toll-free phone line where members can speak with holistic health advisors and medical doctors about their individual health concerns. In addition to its natural product offerings, Life Extension publishes a fantastic monthly magazine. For more information on Life Extension, go to www.lef.org or call 001-1-800-226-2370.

Whole Grains

Just because a bread, cereal or pasta product is brown in colour, don't assume that it is a whole-grain product. Check the ingredient list for the words 'whole grain' or 'whole wheat' to decide if they are made from a whole grain. Some foods are made from a mixture of whole and refined grains.

Some grain products contain significant amounts of bran. Bran provides fibre, which is important for health. However, products with added bran or bran alone (e.g., oat bran) are not necessarily whole-grain products.

On their website, www.wholegrainlife.com, General Mills offers excellent information regarding 'What Is a Whole Grain?' and 'How to Find a Whole Grain Product'. The good news is that General Mills products are readily available in supermarkets across the globe.

Kashi (www.kashi.com) is another of one of my favourite whole-grain brands. I particularly love the Company's logo: '7 whole grains on a mission.' I stock Kashi products in both of my Natural Medicine Stores, but they are also available in the health food or organic food aisle in many stores.

Another brand to check out is Food For Life (www.foodfor life.com). I am a huge fan of their organic sprouted whole-grain pastas and breads. Again, I stock Food for Life products in my Natural Medicine Store, but to find out where you can buy them, check out the website's built-in store finder.

Organic House-Cleaning Products

Remember that it is important to decrease your exposure to environmental oestrogens or xenoestrogens. I recommend using organic house-cleaning products when at all possible. Two good sources for online purchasing are www.heathers naturals.com and www.organiccleaning.com.

Safe Cosmetics

I urge you to make sure that your cosmetics are safe. Many are not. The Campaign for Safe Cosmetics is a coalition of public health, educational, religious, labour, women's, environmental and consumer groups. The coalition's goal is to protect consumer health by requiring the health and beauty industry to phase out the use of chemicals linked to cancer, birth defects and other health problems, and replace them with safer alternatives.

The Safe Cosmetics Campaign began in 2002 with the release of a report, Not Too Pretty: Phthalates, Beauty Products and the FDA. For the report, environmental and public health groups contracted with a laboratory to test seventy-two name-brand, off-the-shelf beauty products for the presence of phthalates, a family of industrial chemicals linked to permanent birth defects in the male reproductive system.

You can find a listing of who has pledged not to use harmful chemicals and to implement substitution plans that replace hazardous materials with safer alternatives in every market they serve on the Safe Cosmetics Campaign website: www.safecosmetics.org/companies/signers.cfm. Several major cosmetics companies, including OPI, Avon, Estee Lauder, L'Oreal, Revlon, Proctor & Gamble and Unilever have thus far refused to sign the Compact for Safe Cosmetics.

The good news is that safe cosmetics are readily available. My co-author Genie James's favourite source for safe or 'green' make-up and hair colour is The Body Shop. *Marketing Week* has reported that The Body Shop was voted the Top Green Brand in the United Kingdom and the eighth-greenest brand in the United States. These findings are according to the recent 2007 Image Power Green Brands Survey and *Marketing Week*/Brand Index Online Survey. You can purchase The Body Shop products online, www.thebodyshop.com, or just head out to your nearest high street branch.

Recently Genie also discovered a delightful website where you can purchase safe cosmetics online. Check out www.themomspa.com.

Water Bottles

As stated in earlier chapters, you should be drinking a lot of water, but please beware of plastic water bottles. Plastics made from polycarbonate resin can leach bisphenol-A (BPA), a potent hormone disruptor. BPA, a chemical found in epoxy resin and polycarbonate plastics, may impair the reproductive organs and have adverse effects on tumours, breast tissue development and prostate development by reducing sperm count.

BPA can leach into water bottles through normal wear and tear and exposure to heat and cleaning agents. This includes leaving your plastic water bottle in your car during errands, in your backpack during hikes and running it through your dishwasher or using harsh detergents. What's more, a 2003 study conducted by the University of Missouri published in the journal *Environmental Health Perspectives* found that detectable levels of BPA leached into liquids at room temperature. This means just having your plastic water bottle sitting on your desk can be potentially harmful. The best thing to do is to avoid plastic altogether. (Side note: Baby bottles made from polycarbonate plastics have quietly disappeared from the market despite industry assurances that polycarbonate plastics are safe.)

There are two approaches to take to avoid exposure to BPA. First, if you are active and take water with you, switch to a stainless steel water bottle. But, be careful. Many products on the market are lined with an epoxy finish. This defeats the purpose. Make sure that the bottle is stainless steel both inside and out. Stainless steel water bottles are light, durable and hold both hot and cold liquids well. My favourite stainless steel water bottle can be found at www.holisticphysician.com/onlinestore/waterfilters/new_wave_enviro/polycarbonate_plastic_containers.htm.

The second approach is to reuse glass containers such as quart-sized juice bottles. Yes, they are a bit heavier but are good solutions if you're in an office environment where mobility isn't an issue. Or you can buy glass water bottles. Check out the following link to Aquasana AQ6000 Glass Water Bottles: www.medmarketplace.com/aquasana-aq6000-glass-water-bottles-set-of-six-29709.html.

Recommended Reading

Books

If you have not already done so, I strongly recommend that you read my first book, *From Hormone Hell to Hormone Well*. In it I provide you with an even stronger foundation regarding the safety and efficacy of bio-identical hormone replacement. You may purchase it on line via my website, www.hormonewell.com, through www.amazon.co.uk or at your local bookstore.

In addition, there are many other physician pioneers and medical experts who have helped lay a foundation of learning and knowledge regarding bio-identical hormone therapy. I have the following books in my personal library. Each author offers the reader the benefit of additional information and another perspective. Please note that these resources are not prioritised by perceived merit but are listed in alphabetical order according to author.

Lee, John R, MD, *Natural Progesterone, The Multiple Role of a Remarkable Hormone.* Sebastopol, CA: BLL Publishing, 1993.

Lee, John R, MD, with Jesse Hanley, MD, and Virginia Hopkins. *What Your Doctor May Not Tell You About Perimenopause.* New York: Warner Books, 1999.

Lee, John R, MD, with Virginia Hopkins. *What Your Doctor May Not Tell You About Menopause.* New York: Warner Books, 1996.

Lee, John R, MD, with David Zava, PhD, and Virginia Hopkins. *What Your Doctor May Not Tell You About Breast Cancer.* New York: Warner Books, 2002.

Northrup, Christiane, MD, *The Wisdom of Menopause: Creating Physical and Emotional Health and Healing During the Change.* New York: Bantam Books, 2001.

Northrup, Christiane, MD, *Women's Bodies, Women's Wisdom: Creating Physical and Emotional Health and Healing.* New York: Bantam Books, 1994.

Schwartz, Erika, MD, *The Hormone Solution.* New York: Warner Books, 2002.

Seaman, Barbara. *The Greatest Experiment Ever Performed on Women: Exploding the Estrogen Myth.* New York: Hyperion Books, 2003.

Shulman, Neil, MD, and Kim S Edmunds, MD, *Healthy Transitions: A Woman's Guide to Perimenopause, Menopause & Beyond.* New York: Prometheus Books, 2004.

Somers, Suzanne, *The Sexy Years, Discover the Hormone Connection: The Secret to Fabulous Sex, Great Health, and Vitality for Women and Men.* New York: Crown Publishers, 2004.

Taylor, Eldred, MD, and Ava Bell-Taylor, MD, *Are Your Hormones Making You Sick?* Physicians Natural Medicine, Inc., 2000.

Whitaker, Julian, MD, *Dr. Whitaker's Guide to Natural Hormone Replacement.* Potomac, MD: Phillips Publishing, 1999.

Wilson, James L, ND, DC, PhD, *Adrenal Fatigue.* Petaluma, CA: Smart Publications, 2003.

Wright, Jonathan V, MD, and John Morgenthaler, *Natural Hormone Replacement for Women Over 45.* Petaluma, CA: Smart Publications, 1997.

Newsletters

E-mail newsletters can be a great source of new information regarding hormone health. They can also serve as excellent reminders of good information you might have read once but have forgotten. There are several excellent newsletters available today. I recommend that you check out and sign up for:

My own. You can register to receive my free monthly newsletter via my website: www.hormonewell.com

Women in Balance: www.womeninbalance.org

Virginia Hopkins' Healthwatch: www.virginiahopkins healthwatch.com

The Natural Progesterone Advisory Network: www. natural-progesterone-advisory-network.com

Best Resource: Yourself

In closing, I want to take a minute to remind each reader that no one can tell you what is right for you, your body or for your health. I encourage you to read, ask questions and do your homework. While it is my privilege to be your resource, when it comes to your health and well being only *you* can be your own final authority.

ABOUT THE AUTHORS

Dr C W Randolph, Jr, is an internationally recognised medical expert in the field of bio-identical hormone replacement, who has successfully treated thousands of women and men with hormone imbalances for more than a decade. He is a board-certified obstetrician and gynaecologist who practiced as a compounding pharmacist before returning to medical school.

Dr Randolph is also the co-founder of The Natural Hormone Institute of America, a Diplomate of the American Board of Holistic Medicine and a member of The International Academy of Compounding Pharmacists.

He continues to be a frequent speaker for medical and women's organisations across the United States and is also the co-author of the bestselling book, *From Hormone Hell to Hormone Well*.

Go to http://hormonewell.com/intertview.html to see Dr Randolph's interview on the *CBS Early Show*.

For more than two decades, **Genie James** has been nationally acknowledged as a change-agent in women's health. In 2004, she co-founded The Natural Hormone Institute of America with CW Randolph, Jr, in order to create a vehicle for getting the word out about the safety and efficacy of bio-identical hormone therapies.

Genie also serves as the executive director of Women Evolving, LLC, an organisation dedicated to educating women how to use their *choice, voice* and *financial power* to enhance their personal health-care while, also, positively impacting our America's overall healthcare delivery system.

In addition to co-authoring *From Hormone Hell to Hormone Well* and *From Belly Fat to Belly Flat* with Dr Randolph, Genie is the author of *Making Managed Care Work* and *Winning in the Women's Healthcare Marketplace*.

REFERENCES

Abdulla, M, and P Gruber. 'Role of Diet Modification in Cancer Prevention.' *Biofactors* 12 (2000): 45–51.

Abraham, G E, and R E Rumley. 'The Role of Nutrition in Managing the Premenstrual Tension Syndromes.' *Journal of Reproductive Medicine* 32 (1987): 405–22.

Alam, I, K Lewis, J W Stephens, and J N Baxter. 'Obesity, Metabolic Syndrome and Sleep Apnoea: All Pro-inflammatory States.' *Obesity Review* 8, no. 2 (2007): 119–27.

Allison, D B, G Gadbury, L G Schwartz, R Murugesan, J L Kraker, S Heshka, K R Fontaine, and S B Heymsfield. 'A Novel Soy-Based Meal Replacement Formula for Weight Loss Among Obese Individuals: A Randomized Controlled Clinical Trial.' *European Journal of Clinical Nutrition* 57 (2003): 514–22.

Angell, M. *The Truth About the Drug Companies.* New York: Random House, 2005.

Ann, N Y. *Mind-Body Medicine: Stress and Its Impact on Overall Health and Longevitiy.* New York: New York Academy of Sciences, 2005.

Appleby, M. 'Why Drinking Water Is Really the Key to Weight Loss.' www.inch-aweigh.com, 2006.

Aronson, D. 'Take the Right Vitamins for You.' *Natural Health* (August 2003): 67–77.

Babal, K. 'Reversing Liver Damage: The Body's Largest Detox Organ Needs Repair Work Now and Then.' *Nutrition Science News* (October 1997).

Balch, J, and P Balch. *Prescription for Nutritional Healing: A-to-Z Guide to Supplements.* Garden City Park, NY: Avery, 1998.

Barbosa, J C, T D Shultz, S J Filley, and D C Neiman. 'The Relationship Among Adiposity, Diet, and Hormone Concentrations in Vegetarian and Nonvegetarian Postmenopausal Women.' *American Journal of Clinical Nutrition* 51 (1990): 798–803.

Barrett-Connor, E, and T L Bush 'Estrogen and Coronary Heart Disease in Women.' *Journal of the American Medical Association* 265 (1991): 1861–67.

Barrett-Connor, E, D Grady, and M L Sefanik. 'The Rise and Fall of Menopausal Hormone Therapy.' *Annual Review of Public Health* 26 (2005): 115–40.

Batterham, Rachel. *Journal of Cell Metabolism* (2006).

Benson, H, and E M Stuart. *The Wellness Book.* New York: Fireside, 1992.

Biskin, M S. 'Nutritional Deficiency in the Etiology of Menorrhagia,

Metrorrhagia, Cystic Mastitis and Premenstrual Tension: Treatment with Vitamin B Complex.' *Journal of Clinical Endocrinology Metabolism* 3 (1943): 227.

Blair, S, H Kohl, R Paffenbarger, D Clark, K Cooper, and L Gibbons. 'Physical Fitness and All-Cause Mortality: A Prospective Study of Healthy Men and Women.' *Journal of the American Medical Association* 262 (1989): 2395–2401.

Blumenthal, J, R Williams, T Needles, and A Wallace. 'Psychological Changes Acompanying Aerobic Exercise in Healthy Middle-Aged Adults.' *Psychosomatic Medicine* 44 (1982): 529–36.

Boggiano, M M, A I Artiga, C E Pritchett, P C Chandler-Laney, M L Smith, and A J Eldridge. 'High Intake of Palatable Food Predicts Binge-Eating Independent of Susceptibility to Obesity: An Animal Model of Lean vs. Obese Binge-Eating and Obesity With and Without Binge-Eating.' *International Journal of Obesity* (2007).

Borysenko, J. *Minding the Body, Mending the Mind.* Reading, MA: Addison-Wesley, 1987.

Campana, W M, and C R Baumrucker. *Handbook of Milk Composition: Hormones and Growth Factors in Bovine Milk.* New York: Academic Press, 1995.

Chang, M L W. 'Dietary Pectic: Effect on Metabolic Processes in Rats.' In *Unconventional Sources of Dietary Fiber,* edited by I. Furda. Washington, DC: American Chemical Society, 1983.

Chen, I, S Safe, and L Bjeldanes. 'Indole-3-Carbinol and Diindolylmethane as Aryl Hydrocarbon Receptor Agonists and Antagonists in T47D Human Breast Cancer Cells.' *Journal of the National Cancer Institute* 7 (1996): 1069–76.

Cho, E J, Y A Lee, H H Yoo, and T Yokozawa. 'Protective Effects of Broccoli Against Oxidative Damage in Vitro and in Vivo.' *Journal of Nutritional Scientific Vitaminology* 52, no. 6 (2006): 437–44.

Colbert, D. *The Bible Cure for Thyroid Disorders.* Lake Mary, FL: Siloam, 2004.

Collins, K. 'How Whole Grains Can Fight Disease.' Available online at www.msnbc.msn.com/id/7080356.

Deibert , P, D Konig, A Schmidt-Trucksaess, K S Zaenker, I Frey, U Landmann, and A Berg. 'Weight Loss Without Losing Muscle Mass in Pre-obese and Obese Subjects Induced by a High-Soy-Protein Diet.' *International Journal of Obesity* 28 (2004): 1349–52.

Diamond, J. *Surviving Male Menopause.* Naperville, IL: Sourcebooks, 2000.

Dossey, L. *Reinventing Medicine: Beyond Mind-Body to a New Era of Healing.* San Francisco: HarperSanFrancisco, 1999.

Dubey, R K, D G Gillespie, E K Jackson, and Paul J Keller. '17B-Estradiol, Its Metabolites, and Progesterone Inhibit Cardiac Fibroblast Growth.' *Hypertension* 31 (1998): 522. Available online at www.ahajournals.org.

Edwards, C. 'Mechanisms of Action on Dietary Fiber on Small Intestinal Absorption and Motility.' In *New Development in Dietary Fiber*. New York: Plenum Press, 1990.

Eisenstein, J, S B Roberts, G Dallal, and E Saltzman. 'Structured Weight-Loss Programs: Meta-Analysis of Weight Loss at 24 Weeks and Assessment of Effects of Intervention Intensity.' *Advanced Therapy* 21 (2004): 61–75.

Elkins, R. *Nature's Phen-Fen: Natural Supplements for Losing Weight*. Pleasant Grove, UT: Woodland Publishing, 1997.

Epstein, S. 'American Beef: Why Is It Banned in Europe?' Available online at http://preventcancer.com/consumers/general/hormones_meat.htm.

Fontaine, K R, D Yang, G L Gadbury, S Heshka, L G Schwartz, R Murugesan, J L Kraker, M Heo, S B Heymsfield, and D B Allison. 'Results of a Soy-Based Meal Replacement Formula on Weight, Anthropometry, Serum Lipids and Blood Pressure During a 40-week Clinical Weight-Loss Trial.' *European Journal of Clinical Nutrition* 57 (2003): 514–22.

Fournier, L R, R Borchers, L M Robison, M Wiediger, J S Park, B P Chew, M K McGuire, D A Sclar, T L Skaer, and K A Beerman. 'The Effects of Soy Milk and Isoflavone Supplements on Cognitive Performance in Healthy, Postmenopausal Women.' *Journal of Nutrition, Health, and Aging* 11, no. 2 (2007): 155–64.

Friel, P N, C Hinchcliffe, and J V Wright. 'Hormone Replacement with Estradiol: Conventional Oral Doses Result in Excessive Exposure to Estrogen.' *Alternative Medical Review* 10 (2005): 36–41.

Fukada,Y, K Kimura, and Y Ayaki. 'Effects of chitosan feeding on intestinal bile acid metabolism in rats.' *Lipids* 20 (1991): 395–99.

Furda, I 'Interaction of Dietary Fiber with Lipids: Mechanic Theories and Their Limitations.' In *New Developments in Dietary Fiber*. New York: Plenum Press, 1990.

Gandhi, R, and S M Snedeker. 'Consumer Concerns About Hormones in Food.' Available online at http://envirocancer.cornell.edu/Factsheet/Diet/fs37.hormones.cfm.

Garry, P J, R N Baumgartner, S G Brodie, G D Montoya, H C Liang, R D Lindeman, and T M Williams. 'Estrogen Replacement Therapy, Serum Lipids, and Polymorphism of the Apolipoprotein E Gene.' *Clinical Chemistry* 45 (1999): 1214–23. Available online at www.Clinichem.org.

Gaudet, T W, P Spencer, and A Weil. *Consciously Female*. New York: Bantam Books, 2004.

Gearon, C J. 'Midlife or Menopause?' Available online at http://health.discovery.com/centers/mens/articles/andropause.html.

Geim, C, U Ehlert, and D H Hellhammer. 'The Potential Role of Hypocortisolism in the Pathophysiology of Stress-Related Bodily Disorders.' *Psychoneuroendocrinology* 25, no. 1 (2000): 1–35.

Giuca, L. 'Nothing Complex About Choosing the Right Carbohydrates in

Diet.' *The Milwaukee Journal Sentinel,* 1999. Available online at www.findarticles.com/p/articles/mi_qn4196/is_19990117/ai_n10494852.

Goldin, B R, H Adlercreutz, J T Dwyer, L Swenson, J H Warram, and S L Gorbach. 'Effect of Diet on Excretion of Estrogens in Peri- and Postmenopausal Women.' *Cancer Research* 14 (1981): 3771–73.

Goldin, B R, and S L Gorbach. 'Effect of Diet on the Plasma Levels, Metabolism, and Excretion of Estrogens.' *American Journal of Clinical Nutrition* 48 (1988): 787–90.

Goldstein, J, C K Sites, and M J Toth. 'Progesterone Stimulates Cardiac Muscle Protein Synthesis via Receptor-Dependent Pathway.' *Fertility and Sterility* 82, no. 2 (2004): 430–36. Available online at www.sciencedirect.com.

Graham, J. 'How Stress Makes You Fat.' *Ladies Home Journal* (July 2005): 168–74.

Greider, K. *The Big Fix.* New York: Public Affairs, 2003.

Grossman, T. *The Baby Boomers' Guide to Living Forever.* Golden, CO: Hubristic Press, 2000.

Hawthorne, F. *Inside the FDA.* Hoboken, NJ: John Wiley & Sons, 2005.

Holm R R, and P Bjorntorp. 'Food-Induced Cortisol Secretion in Relation to Anthropometric, Metabolic and Haemodynamic Variables in Men.' *International Journal of Obesity-Related Metabolic Disorders* 24, no. 4 (2000): 416–22.

Holmes, M. 'Adrenal Fatigue: The Effects of Stress and High Cortisol Levels.' *Women to Women* (2006): 1–4.

Hoy, C. *The Truth About Breast Cancer.* Ontario, Canada: Stoddart, 1996.

Igimi, H, M Nishimura, R Kodama, and H Ide. 'Studies on the Metabolism of d-Limonene: The Absorption, Distribution, and Exvertion of d-Limonene in Rats.' *Xenobiotica* 4, no. 2 (1974): 77–84.

Ikeda, I, M Sugano, K Yoshida, E Sasaki, Y Iwamoto, and K Hatano. 'Effects of Chitosan Hydrolysates on Lipid Absorption and on Serum and Liver Lipid Concentrations in Rats.' *Journal of Agricultural and Food Chemistry* 41 (1993): 431–435.

Ingram, D M, F C Bennett, D Wilcox, and N de Klerk. 'Effect of Low-Fat Diet on Female Sex Hormone Levels.' *Journal of the National Cancer Institute* 79 (1987): 1225–29.

Jenness, R. 'Composition of Milk.' *Fundamentals of Dairy Chemistry,* edited by N. P. Wong, R. Jenness, J. Kenney, and E. H. Marth. New York: Reinhold, 1988.

Jeong, H J, Y G Shin, I H Kim, and J M Pezzuto. 'Inhibition of Aromatase Activity by Flavonoids.' *Archives of Pharmacological Research* 22 (1999): 309–12.

Kannel, W B, M C Hjortland, P M McNamara, and T Gordon. 'Menopause and Risk of Cardiovascular Disease: The Framingham Study.' *Annals of International Medicine* 85 (1976): 447–452.

Kao, Y C, C Zhou, M Sherman, C A Laughton, and S Chen. 'Molecular Basis of the Inhibition of Human Aromatase by Flavone and Isoflavone Phytoestrogens: A Site-Directed Mutagenesis Study.' *Environmental Health Perspectives* 106, no. 2 (1998): 85–92.

Kellis, J T, and L E Vickery. 'Inhibition of Human Estrogen Synthetase by Flavones.' *Science* 225, no. 4666 (1984): 1032–34.

Kelly, J, D Kaufman, K Kelly, L Rosenberg, T Anderson, and A Mitchell. 'Recent Trends in Use of Herbal and Other Natural Products.' *Archives of Internal Medicine* 165, no. 3 (2005). Available online at http://archinte.amaassa.org/cgi/content/abstract/165/3/281.

Keys, A, and M Keys. *How to Eat Well and Stay Well the Mediterranean Way.* Garden City, NY: Doubleday, 1975.

Knorr, D. 'Recovery and Utilization of Chitin and Chitosan in Food Processing Waste Management.' *Food Technology* 45 (1991): 114–22.

Kodama, R, A Okubo, E Araki, K Noda, H Ide, and T Ikeda. 'Studies on the Metabolism of d-Limonene as a Gallstone Solubilizer: Effects on Development of Mouse Fetuses and Offspring.' *Oyo Yakuri* 13, no. 6 (1977): 863–73.

Lee, J R *Natural Progesterone: The Multiple Role of a Remarkable Hormone.* Sebastopol, CA: BLL Publishing, 1993.

Lee, J R, J Hanley, and V Hopkins. *What Your Doctor May Not Tell You About Perimenopause: Balance Your Hormones and Your Life from Thirty to Fifty.* New York: Warner Books, 1999.

Lee, J R, and V Hopkins. *What Your Doctor May Not Tell You About Menopause.* New York: Warner Books, 1996.

Lee, J R, D Zava, and V Hopkins. *What Your Doctor May Not Tell You About Breast Cancer: How Hormone Balance Can Help Save Your Life.* New York: Warner Books, 2002.

Leon, A, J Connett, D Jacobs, and R Rauramaa. 'Leisure-Time Physical Activity Levels and Risk of Coronary Heart Disease and Death: The Multiple Risk Factor Intervention Trial.' *Journal of the American Medical Association* 258 (1987): 2388–95.

Leonetti, H B, S Longo, and J N Anasti. 'Transdermal Progesterone Cream for Vasomotor Symptoms and Postmenopausal Bone Loss.' *Obstretrics and Gynecology* 94 (1999): 225–28.

Lerner, M *Choices in Healing: Integrating the Best of Conventional and Complementary Approaches to Cancer.* Cambridge, MA: MIT Press, 1994.

Lewis, T T, S A. Everson-Rose, B Sternfeld, K Karavolos, D Wesley, and L H Powell. 'Race, Education, and Weight Change in a Briacia Sample of Women at Midlife.' *Archives of Internal Medicine* 165 (2005): 545–51.

Lopez, D, M D Sanchez, W Shea-Eaton, and M P McLean. 'Estrogen Activates the High Density Lipoprotein Receptor Gene via Binding to Estrogen Response Elements and Interaction with Sterol Regulatory Element Binding Protein-1A.' *Endocrinology* 143 (2002): 2155–68.

Maezaki, Y, K Tusuji, Y Nakagawa, Y Kawai, and M Akimoto.

'Hypocholesterolemic Effect of Chitosan in Adult Males.' *Bioscience, Biotechnology and Biochemistry* 57 (1993): 1439–44.

Manson, J E, and S Bassuk. *Hot Flashes, Hormones & Your Health*. New York: McGraw-Hill, 2007.

McKwoen, N M, J B Meigs, S Liu, E Saltzman, P W Wilson, and P F Jacques. 'Carbohydrate Nutrition, Insulin Resistance, and the Prevalence of the Metabolic Syndrome in the Framingham Offspring Cohort.' *Diabetes Care* 27 (2004): 518–46.

Mendelsohn, M E, and R H Karas. 'The Protective Effects of Estrogen on the Cardiovascular System.' *New England Journal of Medicine* 340 (1999): 1801–11.

Miller, V M, D J Tindall, and P Y Liu. 'Of Mice, Men, and Hormones.' *Arteriosclerosis, Thrombosis, and Vascular Biology* 24 (2004): 995.

Morales, A J, R H Hubrich, and J Y Hwang. 'The Effect of Six Months' Treatment with a 100 mg Daily Dose of Dehydroepiandrosterone on Circulating Sex Steroids.' *Clinical Endocrinology* 29 (1998): 421–32.

Morales, A J, J J Nolan, J C Nelson, and S S C Yen. 'Effects of Replacement Dose of DHEA in Men and Women of Advancing Age.' *Journal of Clinical Endocrinology Metabolism* 78 (1994): 1360.

Myers, H F, T T Lewis, and T Parker-Dominguez. *Stress, Coping and Minority Health: Biopsychosocial Perspectives on Ethnic Health Disparities*. Thousand Oaks, CA: Sage Publications, 2003.

Nestler, J E, C O Barlascini, J N Clore, and W G Blackard. 'Dehydroepiandrosterone Reduces Serum Low Density Lipoprotein Levels and Body Fat but Does Not Alter Insulin Sensitivity in Normal Men.' *Journal of Clinical Endocrinology Metabolism* 66 (1988): 57–61.

Nhat, H T, *Being Peace*. Berkeley, CA: Parallaz Press, 1987.

Northrup, C. *The Wisdom of Menopause: Creating Physical and Emotional Health and Healing During the Change*. New York: Bantam, 2001.

Northrup, C. *Women's Bodies, Women's Wisdom: Creating Physical and Emotional Health and Healing*. New York: Bantam Books, 1994.

Opdyke, D J L. 'Monographs on Fragrance Raw Materials.' *Food and Cosmetics* 13 (1975): 825–26.

Park, S J, L T Goldsmith, J H Skurnick, G Weiss, and A Wojtczuk. 'Characteristics of the Urinary Luteinizing Hormone Surge in Young Ovulatory Women.' *Fertility and Sterility* (2007).

Pathak, N, S Khandelwal. 'Role of Oxidative Stress and Apoptosis in Cadmium Induced Thymic Atrophy and Splenomegaly in Mice.' *Toxicology* 169, no. 2 (2007): 95–108.

Pelissero, C, M J Lenczowski, D Chinzi, B Davail-Cuisset, and J P Sumpter. 'Fostier Effects of Flavonoids on Aromatase Activity: An in Vitro Study.' *Journal of Steroidal, Biochemical, and Molecular Biology* 57 (1996): 215–23.

Plechner, A J. 'Cortisol Abnormality as a Cause of Elevated Estrogen and

Immune Destabilization: Insights for Human Medicine from a Veterinary Perspective.' *Medical Hypotheses* 62, no. 4 (2004): 575–81.

Prentice, R, F C Bennett, C Clifford, S Gorbach, B Goldin, and D Byar. 'Dietary Fat Reduction and Plasma Estradiol Concentration in Healthy Postmenopausal Women.' *Journal of the National Cancer Institute* 82 (1990): 129–34.

Purohit, A, H A Hejaz, and L Walden. 'The Effect of 2-Methoxyoestrone-3-O-Sulphamate on the Growth of Breast Cancer Cells and Induced Mammary Tumours.' *International Journal of Cancer* 85 (2000): 584–89.

Raloff, J. 'Hormones in Your Milk.' *Science News Online* 164, no. 18 (2003). Available online at http://sciencenews.org/articles/20031101/food.asp.

Randall, M. 'Hormones and Belly Fat.' Available online at http://abc.net.au/overnights/stories/s1258936.htm.

Randolph, Jr, CW, and G James. *From Hormone Hell to Hormone Well.* Jacksonville Beach, FL: Natural Hormone Institute of America, 2004.

Ray, A, R Semba, J Walston, L Ferrucci, A Cappola, M. Ricks, Q L Xue, and L Fried. 'Low Serum Selenium and Total Carotenoids Predict Mortality Among Older Women Living in the Community: The Women's Health and Aging Studies.' *American Society for Nutrition* 136 (2006): 172–76. Available online at http://jn.nutrition.org/cgi/content/abstract/136/1/172.

Razdan, A, and D Pattersson. 'Effect of Chitin and Chitosan on Nutrient Digestibility and Plasma Lipid Concentrations in Broiler Chickens.' *British Journal of Nutrition* 72 (1994): 277–88.

Reiss, U, and M Zucker. *Natural Hormone Balance for Women.* New York: Pocket Books, 2001.

Remer, T, and F Manz. 'Estimation of the Renal Net Acid Excretion by Adults Consuming Diets Containing Variable Amounts of Protein.' *Amerian Journal of Clinical Nutrition* 59 (1994): 1356–61.

Renland, J G, and P E Johnson. 'Dietary Calcium and Manganese Effects on Menstrual Cycle Symptoms.' *American Journal of Obstetrics and Gynecology* 168 (1993): 141.

Rose, D P, J R Loughridge, C Cohen, and L E Strong. 'Effect of Low-Fat Diet on Female Sex Hormone Levels in Women with Cystic Breast Disease.' *Journal of the National Cancer Institute* 78 (1987): 623–26.

Rowen, R. 'Redesigned Supplement Fights Breast and Prostate Cancer.' *Dr. Robert Jay Rowen's Second Opinion* 15, no. 8 (2005).

Sahelian, R. 'New Supplements and Unknown, Long-Term Consequences.' *American Journal of Natural Medicine* 4 (1997): 8.

Saunders, D. 'A View of the Mediterranean Diet Pyramid.' Available online at www.changingshape.com/resources/articles/the-mediterranean-diet.asp.

Schoppen, B, A Carbajal, A Perez-Granados, F Vivas, and M Vaquero. 'Food, Energy and Macronutrient Intake of Postmenopausal Women from a Menopause Program.' *Nutricion Hospitalaria* 20, no. 2 (2005): 101–9.

Schulze, M B, S Liu, E B Rimm, J E Manson, W C Willett, and F B Hu. 'Glycemic Index, Glycemic Load, and Dietary Fiber Intake and Incidence of Type 2 Diabetes in Younger and Middle-Aged Women.' *American Journal of Clinical Nutrition* 80 (2004): 348–56.

Schwartz, E. *The Hormone Solution.* New York: Warner Books, 2002.

Seaman, B. *The Greatest Experiment Ever Performed on Women: Exploding the Estrogen Myth.* New York: Hyperion Books, 2003.

Shomon, M. 'Do Soy Foods Negatively Affect Your Thyroid?' Available online at http://thyroid-info.com/articles/soydangers.htm.

Shulman, N, and K S Edmunds. *Healthy Transitions: A Woman's Guide to Perimenopause, Menopause & Beyond.* New York: Prometheus Books, 2004.

Shultz, T D, and J E Leklem. 'Nutrient Intake and Hormonal Status of Premenopausal Vegetarian Seventh-Day Adventists and Premenopausal Nonvegetarians.' *Nutrition and Cancer* 4 (1983): 247–59.

Somers, S. *The Sexy Years, Discover the Hormone Connection: The Secret to Fabulous Sex, Great Health, and Vitality for Women and Men.* New York: Crown Publishers, 2004.

Sun, Y, C Gu, X Lui, W Liang, P Yao, J L Bolton, and R B van Breemen. 'Ultrafiltration Tandem Mass Spectrometry of Estrogens for Characterization of Structure and Affinity for Human Estrogen Receptors.' *PubMed Central* 16, no. 2 (2005): 271–79. Available online at www.Pubmedcentral.nih.gov.

Taylor, E B, and A Bell-Taylor. *Are Your Hormones Making You Sick?* Physicians' Natural Medicine, 2000.

Teta, J, and K Teta. 'The Impact of Lifestyle Choices and Hormonal Balance on Coping with Stress.' *The Townsend Letter* (2005).

Trichopoulou, A, T Costacou, C. Bamia, and D Trichopoulou. 'Adherence to a Mediterranean Diet and Survival in a Greek Population.' *The New England Journal of Medicine* 348, no. 26 (2003): 2599-2608.

Tsuji, M, Y Fujisaki, and Y Arikawa. 'Studies on the Metabolism of d-Limonene as a Gallstone Solubilizer: Chronic Toxicity in Rats.' *Oyo Yakuri* 9, no. 3 (1975): 403–412.

Uebelhack, R, J U Blohmer, H J Graubaum, R Busch, J Gruenwald, and K D Wernecke. 'Black Cohosh and St. John's Wort for Climacteric Complaints.' *Obstetrics and Gynecology* 107 (2006): 247–55.

Usiskin, K S, S Butterworth, and J N Clore. 'Lack of Effect of Dehydroepiandrosterone in Obese Men.' *International Journal of Obesity* 14 (1990): 457–63.

Vaillant, G E *Aging Well.* Boston: Little, Brown, 2002.

Van Duyn, M A, and E Pivonka. 'Overview of the Health Benefits of Fruit and Vegetable Consumption for the Dietetics Professional: Selected Literature.' *Journal of the American Dietary Association* 100 (2000): 1511–21.

Weil, A. *Eating Well for Optimum Health: The Essential Guide to Bringing Health and Pleasure Back to Eating.* New York: Quill, 2001.

Whitaker, J. *Dr. Whitaker's Guide to Natural Hormone Replacement.* Potomac, MD: Phillips Publishing, 1999.

Wilson, J L *Adrenal Fatigue.* Petaluma, CA: Smart Publications, 2001.

Wren, B G, K McFarland, and L Edwards. 'Micronised Transdermal Progesterone and Endometria Response.' *Lancet* 354 (1999): 1447–48.

Wright, J V, and J Morgenthaler. *Natural Hormone Replacement for Women Over 45.* Petaluma, CA: Smart Publications, 1997.

Zimecki, M, and M L Kruzel. 'Milk-Derived Proteins and Peptides of Potential Therapeutic and Nutritive Value.' *Journal of Experimental Therapeutics and Oncology* 6, no. 2 (2007): 86–106.

INDEX

Page numbers followed by an *f* or a *t* indicate figures or tables.

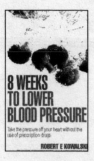
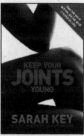